BODY
BUSINESS

Donna Aston grew up in Melbourne, Australia. Fifteen years ago, 20 kg over her present weight, Donna began researching what has become her lifelong passion: health and nutrition. Five years later, she put her knowledge into practice, transforming her body through exercise and diet and going on to represent Australia in numerous international body-shaping competitions. While training and advising clients in Geneva, Switzerland, Donna met her British husband, and she and Adrian now spend much of their time living in Europe. In her personal-training business, Donna has gained a reputation for achieving outstanding results with hundreds of clients, ranging from the 'girl next door' to Australia's celebrities.

Donna's first book, *Fat or Fiction*, was launched in 1999, on her return from representing Australia at the Ms Universe body-shaping competition, and rapidly became an Australian best-seller.

DONNA ASTON

BODY
BUSINESS

VIKING

Viking

Published by the Penguin Group
Penguin Books Australia Ltd
250 Camberwell Road
Camberwell, Victoria 3124, Australia
Penguin Books Ltd
80 Strand, London WC2R 0RL, England
Penguin Putnam Inc.
375 Hudson Street, New York, New York 10014, USA
Penguin Books Canada Limited
10 Alcorn Avenue, Toronto, Ontario, Canada M4V 3B2
Penguin Books (NZ) Ltd
Cnr Rosedale and Airborne Roads, Albany, Auckland, New Zealand
Penguin Books (South Africa) (Pty) Ltd
24 Sturdee Avenue, Rosebank, Johannesburg 2196, South Africa
Penguin Books India (P) Ltd
11, Community Centre, Panchsheel Park, New Delhi 110 017, India

First published by Penguin Books Australia Ltd 2001

7 9 11 13 12 10 8 6

Design by Ellie Exarchos
Typeset in 10.5/17 ITC Legacy Serif Book by Post Pre-press Group, Brisbane, Queensland
Printed and bound in Australia by McPherson's Printing Group, Maryborough, Victoria

National Library of Australia
Cataloguing-in-Publication data:

Aston, Donna.
Body business.

Includes index.
ISBN 0 670 88615 7.

1. Dietetics. 2. Health. 3. Body size. I. Title.

613

www.penguin.com.au

foreword

Donna Aston's personal success story is an inspiration to people who seek to change their body shape and general health.

Donna discovered that the key to successfully changing her body was knowledge. She embarked on a journey designed to learn how her body functioned by seeking out the best information and methods available.

Most women are well aware of the major changes that can occur in their bodies as a result of significant hormonal events such as childbirth or menopause. As the scientific evidence is being pieced together it is becoming clear that hormones mediate major changes in body function.

By understanding how these hormones respond to variations in diet and exercise we can effect changes to our body shape, basal metabolic rate and lean body mass. Even more exciting is the opportunity to reduce the underlying risk of diseases such as heart disease, diabetes and stroke.

It is clear that diet and exercise are powerful tools that can be harnessed to radically reshape our body, improve our health or change our life.

Donna Aston has developed a program that has a sound foundation in medical knowledge and is backed by medical research. Doctors in Australia and around the world have reproduced Donna's personal success in large numbers of patients.

Until recently many medical experts have been critical of diet programs that advocate a reduction in carbohydrate intake. However, the last few years have seen a dramatic change in attitude on the part of some dietary authorities.

Maintaining a healthy lifestyle, reducing weight and minimising body fat are all facilitated by a diet and lifestyle program that acts by influencing the various hormones in the body. I commend Donna Aston's latest diet and health program to you as a practical way to take control of your body and improve your health.

Dr Bruce Farnsworth
Sydney-based consultant gynaecologist
specialising in hormone problems,
bladder problems and bleeding problems

acknowledgements

This book is dedicated to two of the most amazing role models a girl could have: my mum and dad.

To my friend, adviser and brilliant editor of *Fat or Fiction*, Linda Roach – you're the best!

Every book is a lot more than just the writing of its author. I'd like to thank some of the talented people who spent countless hours helping me create this book for you.

Thank you to everyone at Penguin Books Australia for loyally supporting my work. In particular: Clare Forster, my publisher – a true professional; Ellie Exarchos, one of the world's most talented designers – you excelled with *Fat or Fiction* and now you've actually done it again!; Lyn McGaurr – thank you for your patience; Christian Wild – what can I say? a brilliant and creative photographer and a pleasure to work with – thank you again. I'd also like to acknowledge the valuable testimonials kindly submitted by Jane Kennedy and Sigrid Thornton – thank you.

Last, but certainly not least, thank you to my inspirational, brilliant and ever-supportive husband, Adrian.

introduction

For those of you who have not yet read *Fat or Fiction*, I'd better bring you up to date on the evolution of that book, and the continuation of my life-long passion, which has led me to write this sequel. The battle for weight control is a personal one. For several years I was stranded on the dieting merry-go-round, becoming more and more dizzy with confusion (not to mention from lack of food!) and more depressed, as failure after failure after failure only made me fatter.

I tried them all: severe calorie restriction, almost no fat, weird combinations – always followed by overindulgence, endless hours of exercise, magic diet pills, potions and weight-loss products. Obsessed with magazine articles promising me the slim, toned figure that I had longed for, I did what countless thousands of others have done and are still doing: I squandered my hope, my trust and, not least of all, my money!

From this pudgy dieter drowning in the sea of weight-loss myths and hype, I managed to transform myself.

In 1995, I became the first Australian to earn professional status in body-shaping competitions. I have represented Australia in Atlanta, New York and, most recently, at the 1999 Ms Universe Competition in London, in which I came sixth.

After a career of almost thirteen years in personal training, working with hundreds of clients and studying every piece of information I could get my hands on about weight loss and nutrition, I just had to write *Fat or Fiction*. My main goal was to create a way of eating that would provide optimum nutrition and thereby alleviate many of the symptoms that I consider to be related to an unbalanced diet. These include excess body fat/obesity, a suppressed immune system (resulting in recurring viruses etc.), skin problems, diabetes and hundreds of common ailments.

The logic that has inspired me is quite simple. If we are feeding our bodies with the food they need, shouldn't we be able to achieve all of these results with just one eating plan? If your body is functioning at its optimum level in every way, it is quite brilliant and often capable of alleviating all of these symptoms, given the right *fuel*. I analysed many diet and so-called health books prior to writing mine. I searched endlessly for a plan that took a holistic approach to health and nutrition. Much to my amazement, I didn't find one! Hence *Fat or Fiction*.

I knew that *Fat or Fiction* was capable of providing women and men with the bodies that they had always wanted. However, I wasn't prepared for the vast amount of feedback and the myriad requests for more: more information, more structure, more recipes, more on exercise – more, more, more! And so *Body Business* was born.

This book not only expands on *Fat or Fiction* but also goes back to basics, providing structured eating and exercise programs, menu planners and shopping guides. Although it builds upon the foundation established in *Fat or Fiction*, *Body Business* is entirely self-contained and reiterates all essential information.

One concern I have is that some people have pigeon-holed *Fat or Fiction* with diet books that recommend too much protein and too little carbohydrate. Firstly, the very words 'high' and 'low' are deceptive. What is a *high*-protein diet? Is it considered high protein because it is *higher* in protein than the diets many of us are already consuming? To me, 'high protein' means more protein than we actually need, just as 'low carbohydrate' means less carbohydrate than we need. My eating plan probably does consist of more protein and less carbohydrate than you are currently consuming, but that is only because at present you are likely to be eating far too many 'empty' carbohydrates and not nearly enough protein.

I believe that there *are* diets that are too high in protein and too low in carbohydrate and that these *are* extreme. I also believe that, at the other end of the spectrum, the traditional food pyramid is just as extreme. My focus is on balance: *adequate* quantities of protein, carbohydrate and fat.

Is your body in the shape you know is best for you? If the answer is no, try this program; what have you got to lose except some fat?

it worked for me!

I sought Donna out after reading her first book, *Fat or Fiction*, which was such a straightforward and commonsense read that I was interested to meet its author.

We went on to work together as trainer and trainee, and as a student of Donna's I discovered she is a gifted teacher. She has such a wealth of knowledge about health, diet and exercise, but what really sets her apart is her integrity – her altruistic desire to impart her message. She genuinely believes that she has the answer for a better body. And, what's more, she actually does!

Donna has greatly improved my understanding of my own body and how easily I'm able to take care of it. Having the information I need has motivated me to take the necessary steps towards better health and fitness. Donna's first book has been an inspiration to so many people, myself included, and I know this one will give us all an even greater understanding of why her program is so effective.

Sigrid Thornton
actress

Having followed the lifestyle and eating program devised by Donna Aston for a number of years, I can safely say this is the only way I have been able to maintain a healthy weight and body-fat ratio.

I know this philosophy may not be for everyone, but it works for me. I have recommended Donna's book to friends and have watched as the weight has fallen off them. You may find it tough at first because we usually eat so many carbohydrates in our daily diet. However, I've been able to devise my own recipes focusing on fresh, tasty, satisfying unprocessed foods while managing to live without lashings of bread, pasta and potatoes. I also realise that you cannot rely on an eating regimen alone; exercise is absolutely essential, but that can simply translate into a forty-minute walk three times a week, which is, of course, just as important for the soul as it is for the behind!

Jane Kennedy
film and television writer,
performer and producer
Working Dog Productions

I hate to say it, but I was your typical dieter: I'd lose a couple of kilos to fit into that outfit, put them (and maybe one of their buddies) back on, lose a couple more, and so on.

At my first editorial meeting with Donna Aston, however, she suggested I try her program. I was on the low-fat kick at the time. You know the one: white bread, pasta and rice, with very little protein and tiny little meals. I went, cold turkey (yum), to no white food, no sugar, and to dinners so large that my boys were convinced I would balloon into the Michelin man and float away.

After one month I had lost 6 kg of fat and made 2 kg of muscle (Donna had me on a light weights program, and I had always done regular exercise). This weight loss continued, although at a slower pace, and I started feeling full of energy and wellbeing. At the risk of sounding like one of those commercials, my friends began commenting that my body was looking a lot better.

My husband and I still follow Donna's program (although we now have the occasional piece of bread), and it is the best thing we have ever done for our health.

I have never met a more focused, disciplined, committed individual than Donna. And nobody before her had answered my questions concerning both diet and exercise in such a logical, knowledgeable way. Her thirst for the best information about nutrition and weight loss has given her a formidable body of knowledge (not to mention a formidable body!).

One of the most frequent responses to *Fat or Fiction* that I have heard is that it is unpretentious, easy to read and understand, and written with a sense of fun. I have come to know Donna, and I have absolute confidence that *Body Business* will give as much to you and me as *Fat or Fiction*.

Linda Roach
editor
Fat or Fiction

contents

partone

a user's manual

1

chapterone

WHO WILL BENEFIT
FROM THIS EATING PLAN?

You tell me

There does seem to be an endless stream of diet-related books on the market today. Where should we start if we want to educate ourselves on this subject? Which books are worth reading and which are simply trying to sell us yet another gimmick?

Many publications about diet are financed or subsidised in some way by companies that have a vested interest in promoting a particular way of eating. Whether they are breakfast-food con-glomerates or weight-loss companies, the effect of their backing can be quite insidious. I do not represent a cereal company or any other organisation wishing to sell you a diet product. Unlike the countless weight-loss clinics out there, my aim is to help you become completely independent and self-motivated. Many weight-loss programs want you to become totally reliant on their services and sometimes even their food products. When, inevitably, you regain that weight, back you go – over and over again. I'm simply a former yo-yo dieter who has spent more than ten years researching this subject, and I believe I have developed something unique. You don't need all those fancy products and potions. You need to gain enough knowledge to be confident. The success you will have as soon as you start my program will allow you the freedom to live a healthy, *slim* lifestyle, without the torture, stress and complication of calorie restriction and deprivation.

IS THIS BOOK FOR YOU?

Circle the appropriate numbers beneath your answers in the quiz below.

QUIZ	YES	SOMETIMES/ MAYBE	NO
1 Do you find yourself helpless at the thought of a Tim Tam, or salivating at the mere mention of a croissant?	3	2	1
2 Have you made more than three attempts to lose weight?	3	2	1
3 Do you consider yourself a yo-yo dieter?	3	2	1
4 Have you ever purchased creams or pills that claimed to help you lose weight/tone up?	3	2	1
5 Does your work/lifestyle usually get in the way when you try to commit yourself to exercise and/or new diet plans?	3	2	1
6 Do you have designated 'fat' and 'skinny' clothes in your wardrobe?	3	2	1
7 Do you have a strong desire to improve your body/health yet find it difficult to stay motivated long enough to get results?	3	2	1
8 Does your very existence seem to revolve around food?	3	2	1
9 Have you ever considered resorting to medical/surgical methods of weight loss (e.g. appetite suppressants, liposuction)?	3	2	1
10 Does a lack of confidence in your nutritional knowledge prevent you from structuring your own eating plan?	3	2	1

Now, add the circled numbers to reveal your score.

Between 20 and 30 If your score is within this range, you'd better read on! You are in desperate need of a total lifestyle overhaul.

Between 10 and 20 There is definitely something in this book for you. It sounds as though you *almost* have your head around this 'diet thing' but still need a hand. You have strong willpower, but that's the hard way. It's much easier to take your focus off food by eating the right foods. Relying on willpower is hard – and you know what happens sooner or later . . .

Score of below 10 Well, you're perfect! Put down the book. You and your halo may leave the room.

QUESTION *Is this plan suitable for men, or is it aimed specifically at women?*

ANSWER I can really sum up the answer to this question in one sentence: if you are human, you can benefit from the principles in this book.

Most men love this eating plan because it includes one of their favourite foods: meat! That's right: not rice crackers and a cup of low-fat soup for lunch, but *real food* and plenty of it.

I'm sure that many books published on the subject of diet and nutrition are bought by women, so I guess those publications are marketed with that readership in mind. This does not mean that they are strictly for women though. Men, women and children obviously have varying requirements, depending on body size and composition, activity levels, lifestyle, goals etc. However, the fact remains that all healthy digestive tracts work the same way. We all require the same nutrients but in varying quantities. Nobody's health has ever suffered from their eating a nutritious, balanced diet of 'real food'. I have taken various body sizes into consideration in later chapters to assist you in choosing the most appropriate menu plan.

What about vegetarians? Do you have to eat meat to follow these principles effectively?

'Vegetarian' is a very broad term generally used to describe a diet devoid of most flesh or other products derived from animals.

A 'vegan' is a vegetarian who consumes absolutely no animal products. Less strict vegetarians may eat certain animal-based products (e.g. eggs and dairy products) but exclude flesh (beef, chicken and fish). If your reason for deciding to follow a vegetarian diet is political or has grown out of a concern for animal rights, I respect and accept your right to make that choice. However, if the decision is made in the belief that it will improve health or result in weight loss, then I disagree with it entirely.

If, as a vegetarian, you consume eggs and dairy products, your diet is quite flexible, and it will be easy for you to achieve a nutritional balance. If you are a strict vegan, you will find it more difficult to increase your consumption of protein. Contrary to popular belief, being a vegetarian does not mean that one simply excludes all meat from the diet; cutting out animal protein without substituting other sources of protein creates an unhealthy imbalance of nutrients. Certain food combinations will provide the body with adequate quantities of all necessary amino acids (which are found in protein) and other essential nutrients. This does require a great deal of careful planning and extensive knowledge of food composition and your requirements.

My recommendation for vegans is to acknowledge the main emphasis of this book, which is to establish a healthy lifestyle, taking into account information about anti-oxidants, exercise and the body's requirements for macronutrients (protein, carbohydrates and fats). Regardless of whether you are a vegan or a carnivore, gaining a sound knowledge of the body you will live in for the duration of your life has to be a worthwhile exercise.

2

chaptertwo

BODY COMPOSITION

*Sugar and spice . . . or puppy dogs' tails:
what is your body made of?*

B ody composition refers to how much of your total weight is fat and how much is lean tissue, and you can have this assessed at health and fitness centres or by your doctor. Lean tissue is everything other than stored body fat. Your lean body weight (LBW) is your weight on the scales minus your body fat (see example on page 31).

BODY FAT

The volume of adipose tissue, or body fat, in the human body ranges from 5 to 60 per cent. It is composed of around 80 to 85 per cent fats, 2 per cent protein and 10 per cent water. Your body has built-in storage tanks (fat cells) to accommodate any excess energy food you may consume – a sort of 'spill-over' device. When you tilt the energy-balance equation too far your fat cells take up the slack. If you consume too much energy for your immediate requirements, the leftover is directed to your fat cells, ensuring you will have a reserve fuel supply in the event of the energy balance being tilted the opposite way.

Unlike lean tissue, body fat requires no energy to maintain it. There are several different types of stored fat:

visceral fat fat that accumulates around the internal organs as opposed to directly beneath the skin

abdominal fat visceral fat that accumulates around the abdomen

brown fat a type of fat that stimulates the burning of white fat for energy production

subcutaneous fat fat residing immediately under the dermis of the skin

cellulite a commonly used term for subcutaneous fat, usually around the thighs and hips of women

femoral fat fat that accumulates around the hips and thighs

white adipose fat all adipose tissue other than brown fat.

LEAN TISSUE

Lean tissue does require energy (fuel) to maintain it. In your body, fuel is supplied by the food you consume. Now you can see where the common saying 'you are what you eat' came from. Your lean tissue requires certain kinds of fuel and a particular number of calories for maintenance. Your basal metabolic rate (BMR) defines the energy that is necessary for the basic maintenance of your body. This includes energy used to sustain the movement of involuntary muscles such as the heart and lungs, for synthesis of new protein and to maintain your core temperature.

> This explains why body composition is a crucial element in health and weight loss, and your weight as indicated by the bathroom scales alone is not!

From the information above, I'm sure you have already surmised that the lower your percentage of body fat and the higher your percentage of lean tissue, the healthier and leaner you will be. When you don't have to carry around excess weight in the form of body fat, you will undoubtedly have much more energy. With a higher level of lean tissue, you will not only look toned and well-proportioned, but you will also be able to consume more food than ever before without gaining excess body fat. What a fabulous bonus!

Well, this all sounds perfectly logical in theory, but how do you make it work for you? Read on: the following chapters are going to take you through your own personal transformation, step by step. By the end of this book, you will have all the tools you need to create the results you desire.

The following table rates body-fat percentages according to age and gender.

BODY-FAT PERCENTAGES

AGE	MALES				FEMALES			
	EXCELLENT	GOOD	FAIR	POOR	EXCELLENT	GOOD	FAIR	POOR
20–24	10.8	14.9	19.0	23.3+	18.9	22.1	25.0	29.6+
25–29	12.8	16.5	20.3	24.3+	18.9	22.0	25.4	29.8+
30–34	14.5	18.0	21.5	25.2+	19.7	22.7	26.4	30.5+
35–39	16.1	19.3	22.6	26.1+	21.0	24.0	27.7	31.5+
40–44	17.5	20.5	23.6	26.9+	22.6	26.5	29.3	32.8+
45–49	18.6	21.5	24.5	27.6+	24.3	27.3	30.9	34.1+
50–54	19.5	22.3	25.2	28.3+	25.8	28.9	32.3	35.5+
55–59	20.0	22.9	25.9	28.9+	27.0	30.2	33.5	36.7+
60+	20.3	23.4	26.4	29.5+	27.6	30.9	34.2	37.7+

Excellent This is an above-average rating, showing quite low levels of body fat and perfectly adequate lean tissue. It is a definite advantage for optimum health and wellbeing.

Good If you fall within this range, your body is still in very good condition.

Fair You're slipping. Take care, and re-evaluate your current diet and exercise regimen – it needs some tweaking.

Poor Apart from feeling pretty ordinary, you are also putting your health at risk with this body-fat percentage. Time for a change.

case study jenny

It had always been Jenny's understanding that if she lost enough weight, as measured by her bathroom scales, she would eventually achieve the lean, toned body she desired. After years of dieting as a slightly chubby teenager, Jenny discovered that the battle proved a little more difficult with every passing year.

At twenty-nine years old, Jenny was puzzled, to say the least, to find that her body fat was 39 per cent, even at her 'ideal' weight. With her past dietary habits, she risked compromising her health just to maintain this body composition. Jenny was persevering with the frustration of consuming inadequate calories and nourishment to achieve nothing other than maintenance. Within six weeks of following *Fat or Fiction* principles, Jenny had maintained her weight as measured by the scales, yet her body fat was down to 32 per cent. This was achieved while eating more calories than her previous diet had allowed. Obviously, one of the greatest advantages Jenny has acknowledged is that she doesn't feel hungry all the time. Being hungry for any length of time was stressful, making her feel lethargic and irritable. Jenny is already fitting into her clothes more comfortably, her skin has improved dramatically and her body is taking on a totally new look. By the time she reaches her goal of 24 per cent body fat, Jenny says she'll feel like Wonderwoman.

QUESTION *My body fat was measured at almost 40 per cent. However, I'm only a size 8. How can this be?*

ANSWER To begin with, let's talk about what is a statistically 'normal' range of body fat. Women will always have a higher body-fat percentage than men, due to our wonderful childbearing bodies! Statistics indicate that a healthy range of body fat for women is between 18 and 28 per cent. For men, it is more like between 12 and 18 per cent. If the obesity statistics worldwide were determined by accurate calculations of body composition, I'm sure they would indicate that much more than the estimated 50 per cent of the population was obese. In my own experience of measuring body composition, the majority of women and men have much more than 30 per cent body fat.

In answer to the question above, you do not have to be overweight to be overfat. In other words, you can be small in stature/size, yet your body can still be composed of very little lean tissue and a lot of fat. To use an analogy, look at the measurement of gold. A gold ring can be nine carat, eighteen carat or twenty-four carat yet remain the same size. The only difference is the ratio of gold to other metals, just like our ratio of fat to lean tissue. A *small* body is not necessarily a *lean* body, just as a *larger* body is not necessarily one that is *overfat*. You can manipulate your ratio of fat to lean tissue to achieve a healthy, toned body.

QUESTION   *If I increase my lean weight in an attempt to reduce my body-fat percentage, won't I begin to look too muscular or big?*

ANSWER   Gaining lean tissue and losing body fat does not necessarily mean that you will become bigger, or even change your weight on the scales. If you have less muscle than you need to achieve an optimum ratio of fat to lean tissue, then I can't imagine that you will make excessive gains, particularly if this is not your intention. The weight of your lean tissue may increase with a change in your diet alone, or it may require some form of resistance exercise (such as weight training). Either way, it is very difficult to increase quality lean tissue, let alone have too much of it. It's almost like saying, 'I am working to earn money, but what happens if I earn too much?' As your body fat decreases in volume, you will also be losing fat that is marbled throughout muscle tissue, creating smaller, more compact yet dense muscle tissue that may weigh more. If, heaven forbid, you do find yourself looking too muscular, just cut back on the weight training and watch your muscle deteriorate rapidly. On women, a smooth, thin layer of body fat over toned muscle will appear shapely and firm. Men's hormones enable them to be much harder and leaner than women, but I have met very few women who desire a *hard* look anyway.

FOR YOUR INFORMATION

The body mass index (BMI) is a simple form of measurement often used to determine the physical condition of a person. Although less accurate than an actual body-composition test, it gives a general estimate of how Australians measure up. I can't even begin to imagine what the statistics would be if accurate body-composition testing was used. There are many people out there who are not overweight according to their scales but are certainly outside the healthy range of body-fat levels.

BMI is calculated by dividing our weight in kilograms by the square of our height in metres. In the Australian Bureau of Statistics (ABS) study *How Australians Measure Up*, the BMI of Australian men and women was measured, then put into the categories below.

Less than 20 underweight
20 to less than 25 acceptable
25 to less than 30 overweight
30 or more obese

The ABS has expressed concern that the results of many popular surveys based on self-reported height and weight statistics may be less accurate than results obtained by using the more costly measured method. The BMI of Australians indicates that we are much fatter than we think. The graph below shows the *actual* BMI, calculated using precise measurements.

AUSTRALIAN BODY MASS INDEX

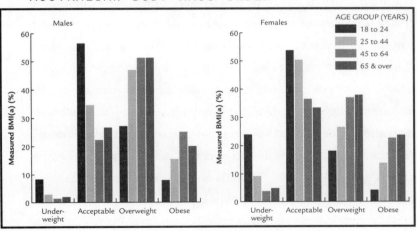

Chart created using figures from *How Australians Measure Up*, Australian Bureau of Statistics, cat. No. 4359.0

SHEDDING SOME LIGHT ON THE YO-YO SYNDROME

Many people assume that exercising will prevent them from losing lean tissue, regardless of their dietary intake. When we exercise, we break down muscle tissue in the process. Muscle tissue is then repaired by the body, gradually improving density and tone and therefore becoming more tolerant of subsequent exercise sessions. Your miraculous body takes care of all this. That is, until you decide to undernourish yourself, creating a deficit of 'tools' with which your body can rebuild and repair itself. If you are exercising, there is a greater demand for a consistent supply of nourishment. If this demand is not met, even temporarily, your body is not capable of adequate repair and muscle tissue is lost. As we now know, the consequence is a lower metabolic rate, which is the very *essence* of the yo-yo syndrome. In a nutshell: exercise will not counteract the yo-yo syndrome and even has the potential to exacerbate its negative effects.

Reducing your calorie intake to a level below that required to maintain your existing BMR is at the very core of yo-yo dieting. So few calories cannot meet your nutritional requirements. The reason we eat food is to gain nourishment to fuel our body and keep it healthy. If we restrict this nourishment by reducing calories too much and by failing to consume good-quality calories, our health will eventually suffer. Many younger people don't give much consideration to health and wellbeing. Appearance alone is commonly their priority. In our teens and twenties, we all think we're invincible. Beginning to witness ageing and deterioration first hand in our thirties can be a rude awakening.

Of course calorie restriction can be considered if you are consuming too many calories to begin with. However, in many instances this is not the case.

There are two basic rules you should follow to avoid, or escape from, the yo-yo syndrome.

• *Never* consume fewer calories than your BMR requires or you will risk losing lean tissue, slowing down your metabolism and jeopardising your health and wellbeing.

• *Always* make sure that the calories you are consuming are of the highest quality. If you can gain the highest possible value from the food you eat, you won't need to overeat to keep hunger at bay.

I had a very young girl come to see me at my consulting rooms soon after reading *Fat or Fiction*. She had been depriving herself of sufficient calories on and off for such a long time that she no longer had any perception of what a 'normal' person would eat in a day. Because she was living away from home while studying, she made a special trip back to visit her mother. She considered her mother to have quite 'normal' eating habits, so she stayed with her for a few weeks to get an idea of how much and how frequently a 'normal' person eats. It was almost as if she had been abducted by aliens and had been living on another planet. How does such a bright young person fall into this vicious cycle? There are many of you out there. I have had literally hundreds of letters, emails and telephone calls from readers who say, 'I've read your book and I love it. It makes so much sense to me. Now where do I start? I need to be told *exactly* what to eat!'

It seems we have become so caught up on this merry-go-round that we no longer have the confidence to listen to our bodies and trust in our choices.

HAVE WE ALL
GONE MAD?

the quick fix

Liposuction? What are we doing? I know a doctor whose speciality is performing liposuction. We have had many in-depth discussions on this subject. He has given me his sales pitch: 'Well, it's really for those people who have tried *everything* and can't shift the fat!' When he realised that I wasn't going to fall for this one, he decided to readily admit that he was 'just doing what people asked for'. You see, we justify it with, 'I've tried everything else, but nothing works.' I've known people who have resorted to liposuction thinking it was the easy way out. They have continued to consume all the wrong foods after surgery, only to regain the weight with a vengeance. You will be told that the fat cells removed cannot return. What you are not told is that fat cells have an ability to e-x-p-a-n-d beyond your wildest dreams. Fat cells are quite accommodating little devils, as many obese people have proved to us all. They have an amazing capacity to grow on demand. Or perhaps your body will just store your excess fat in fat cells elsewhere on your body. Either way, liposuction is not the ideal solution you were searching for, is it? A girl I know decided to have liposuction on her bottom, hips, inner and outer thighs, knees and ankles. She had a total of 2 kg of fat removed. She was promptly wrapped up in a tight, girdle-like bandage, which she was instructed to wear for six weeks after leaving hospital. She had to rest for some time afterwards. After all, she had endured quite major surgery. During her time of rest and recuperation, she gained 9.5 kg. Now, if you do the maths, you will realise that she actually came out of this procedure 7.5 kg heavier, due to the period of compulsory inactivity after surgery. Whoops.

3

chapterthree

EXERCISE

Addressing the flip side of the equation:
how much energy we burn

At its simplest, my philosophy on exercise has always been *just move*. Exercise need not be any more structured than that. However, *Fat or Fiction* has motivated many of you to want to do more, so I will provide you with a specific and comprehensive structure.

Obviously, what is an appropriate exercise plan for each of us is influenced by individual differences, from our physical capabilities to our general desire (or lack of it) to make the time commitment necessary to create an active lifestyle. I have combined my personal-training knowledge with relevant BMR calculations and have individualised, as much as one can in a book, a program for each of you.

In this chapter I explain how to stick to an exercise regimen, what sort of exercise we should undertake and how much energy various activities burn. I also explain what other factors influence the amount of energy we require.

THE GOLDEN RULES OF ESTABLISHING
A PERSONAL EXERCISE ROUTINE

There are certain rules you must follow if you expect to stick to any exercise regimen.

• Choose activities that you enjoy, and *make the time* to pursue them. (Notice I didn't say 'find the time' . . . *big* difference.)

• Make health and exercise higher priorities.

• Be flexible. If your chosen activity is outdoors and it happens to be the middle of winter, have a backup plan. When I was preparing for the 1999 Ms Universe competition, I trained right through Melbourne's winter. My chosen activity was walking – preferably outdoors. Friends would say to me, 'You're not walking today are you? It's pouring!' My answer was always, 'That's what umbrellas are for!' The competitive side of me would rear its head on these occasions. I couldn't get up in front of a judging panel and say, 'Sorry I'm still a little out of shape – it was raining.' However, without such strong motivation I might have needed a backup plan.

• Always make your goals realistic and achievable. Never set a goal that is miles out of your reach. If you are a beginner, you may want to consider setting several small milestones over a period of time rather than aiming at the outset for your *ultimate goal*, which might seem very distant.

• Start off slowly and gradually build up to a higher level. Don't push yourself beyond your limits just to keep up with a friend or class. Your fitness will improve in due time, and when it does you'll find it quite a motivating achievement. If you feel that you need additional advice to get you going, then I recommend you employ the services of a professional (personal trainer, coach).

After assessing the chart on page 26 you may evaluate goals a little differently. It is designed to establish whether your exercise commitments realistically coincide with what you're trying to achieve. The bottom line? *What it takes to achieve your goals.*

> All of the exercise plans in this chapter are recommended on the assumption that you have no major health problems or injuries. If you are taking medication, or have a disease or disability of any kind, please consult a health professional prior to introducing any change in your activity levels and diet.

HOW MANY CALORIES DO YOU BURN?

Establish your body composition then use the chart on page 26 to find out how much energy you are likely to burn during various activities. It's all very well to know how many calories/kilojoules you're eating, but how many do you burn over and above your BMR?

MAKING THIS PLAN WORK FOR YOU

I recommend various types of exercise, which I have set out for you in a simple chart format on pages 24 and 25.

Light cardiovascular exercise slow walking (3–4 km/h), gentle cycling on flat terrain, golf, horse riding, leisurely ice-skating or rollerblading, light housework, recreational swimming.

Moderate cardiovascular exercise brisk walking (6–7 km/h), moderate cycling, tennis, football, volleyball, basketball, swimming (more intensely), snow skiing or waterskiing, mowing grass.

EXERCISE REQUIREMENTS: MALE

BODY COMPOSITION	REALISTIC GOAL*	EXERCISE REQUIREMENTS†	DURATION
Body fat: 36% and over			
Age: under 29 years	under 20% in 8–10 months	light cardiovascular – 7 days per week	30 minutes or 2 × 15 minutes
30–39 years	under 23% in 8–10 months	light resistance training – 2 days per week	45 minutes per session
40–49 years	under 25% in 10 months		total time commitment:
over 50 years	under 25% in 12 months		5 hours per week
Body fat: 25–35%			
Age: under 29 years	18% in 7–8 months	cardiovascular – 7 days per week	40 minutes or 2 × 20 minutes
30–39 years	19% in 7–8 months	(alternate light and moderate)	40 minutes per session
40–49 years	20% in 8–9 months	moderate resistance training – 3 days per week	total time commitment:
over 50 years	22% in 9 months		6 hours 40 minutes per week
Body fat: 18–24%			
Age: under 29 years	15% in 6–7 months	moderate cardiovascular – 7 days per week	45 minutes or 20 and 25 minutes
30–39 years	16% in 6–7 months	resistance training – 4 days per week	1 hour per session
40–49 years	17% in 6–7 months	(alternate moderate and advanced)	total time commitment:
over 50 years	17% in 7 months		9 hours 15 minutes per week
Body fat: under 18%‡			
Age: under 29 years	13% in 4 months	advanced cardiovascular training – 7 days per week	90 minutes or 2 × 45 minutes
30–39 years	14% in 4 months	advanced resistance training – 3–4 days per week	1 hour per session
40–49 years	15% in 4 months		total time commitment:
over 50 years	16% in 5 months		13–14 hours 30 minutes per week

*The 'realistic-goal' figures are based on the higher end of the body-fat scale. If you are at the lower end, less time will be needed to achieve results. These figures are only estimates. Keep in mind that other factors may influence your rate of progress.

† I recommend that you have a thorough medical examination before you start following this program.

‡ If you are in this range, it's highly likely that you are already following an exercise program. Although no changes are necessary, I have listed approximate activity levels required to achieve or maintain this low level of body fat.

EXERCISE REQUIREMENTS: FEMALE

BODY COMPOSITION	REALISTIC GOAL*	EXERCISE REQUIREMENTS†	DURATION
Body fat: 30% and over			
Age: under 29 years	under 25% in 8–10 months	light cardiovascular – 7 days per week	30 minutes or 2 × 15 minutes
30–39 years	under 27% in 8–10 months	light resistance training – twice per week	45 minutes per session
40–49 years	under 27% in 10 months		total time commitment:
over 50 years	under 28% in 10–12 months		5 hours per week
Body fat: 25–29%			
Age: under 29 years	22% in 5 months	cardiovascular – 7 days per week (alternate light with moderate)	40 minutes or 2 × 20 minutes
30–39 years	22% in 5 months	light resistance training – twice per week	45 minutes per session
40–49 years	23% in 5 months		total time commitment:
over 50 years	24% in 5 months although current range is okay		6 hours 10 minutes per week
Body fat: 20–24%‡			
Age: under 29 years	18% in 2 months	cardiovascular – 7 days per week (alternate moderate with advanced)	45 minutes or 20 and 25 minutes
30–39 years	19% in 2 months	moderate resistance training – 3 times per week	1 hour per session
40–49 years	19% in 2 months		total time commitment:
over 50 years	no change recommended		8 hours 15 minutes per week
Body fat: 15–19%§			
Age: under 29 years	no change recommended	advanced cardiovascular training – 7 days per week	1 hour–90 minutes or 2 × 30–45 minutes
30–39 years	" " " "	moderate to advanced resistance training – 3–4 times per week	1 hour per session
40–49 years	" " " "		total time commitment:
over 50 years	" " " "		10–14 hours 30 minutes per week

*The 'realistic-goal' figures are based on the higher end of the body-fat scale. If you are at the lower end, less time will be needed to achieve results. These figures are only estimates. Keep in mind that other factors may influence your rate of progress.

† I recommend that you have a thorough medical examination before you start following this program.

‡ This is a healthy range to be in. It is not necessary to reduce body fat for health improvement.

§ If you are in this range, it's highly likely that you are already following an exercise program. Although no changes are necessary, I have listed approximate activity levels required to achieve or maintain this low level of body fat.

APPROXIMATE CALORIES BURNED DURING ONE HOUR OF ACTIVITY

ACTIVITY	LEAN BODY WEIGHT (KG)												
	35	40	45	50	55	60	65	70	75	80	85	90	95
Sleeping	45	52	58	65	71	78	84	91	97	104	110	117	123
Sitting at a desk	67	78	87	97	106	117	126	136	145	156	165	175	184
Standing/ironing	67	78	87	97	106	117	126	136	145	156	165	175	184
Driving	67	78	87	97	106	117	126	136	145	156	165	175	184
Washing windows	128	147	165	185	202	221	238	258	275	295	312	332	349
Mowing lawns	128	147	165	185	202	221	238	258	275	295	312	332	349
Walking (4 km/h)	110	127	142	159	174	191	206	223	238	255	269	287	301
Walking (6 km/h)	211	244	273	305	334	367	395	428	456	489	517	550	578
Jogging (9 km/h)	328	380	423	474	518	569	613	664	708	759	803	854	898
Cycling (21 km/h)	328	380	423	474	518	569	613	664	708	759	803	854	898
Running (11 km/h)	423	489	545	611	667	733	790	855	912	978	1034	1100	1156
Squash	423	489	545	611	667	733	790	855	912	978	1034	1100	1156
Tennis/Skiing	202	234	261	292	319	351	378	409	436	360	495	526	553
Weeding	202	234	261	292	319	351	378	409	436	360	495	526	553
Swimming (crawl)	180	208	232	260	284	312	336	364	388	416	440	468	492
Weight training (moderate)	270	312	348	390	426	468	504	546	582	624	660	702	738

Advanced cardiovascular exercise jogging or running (8–9 km/h or more), various competitive sports, skipping rope, boxing, squash, cycling uphill, advanced aerobic or spinning classes.

Resistance training Using weights for resistance, either in the gymnasium, at home or in other activities, such as heavy physical labour or other sporting activity. Some sports are considered as anaerobic, or resistance-style, training. These include weight training or power-lifting, gymnastics, some forms of martial arts and self-defence, and yoga. I consider resistance training to be *any activity requiring physical strength*.

The aim of resistance training is to increase and/or maintain lean tissue, thereby reshaping your body, changing its composition and protecting it against injury and deterioration. Whether the exercise you choose is considered light, moderate or advanced depends on the levels of intensity and resistance used.

If you are a beginner, I recommend you seek professional tuition.

case study michael

At our first meeting, 35-year-old Michael entered the room in quite a state. I think he had been psyching himself up in preparation for the severe 'talking to' he expected from me in response to his 42 per cent body fat. He blurted out, 'I'm not giving up any of my wine and social dinners. I enjoy them and they are part of my life, so don't expect me to just give them up – I won't.'

I acknowledged that these issues were important to him, and we continued to discuss his health and weight-loss goals. He was interested in pursuing an exercise program to help him shed the weight and regain some of his former energy. This seemed to be something he could relate to, so we established a gym program for him to start immediately.

As the weeks passed I saw Michael regularly to monitor his progress. Initially, without dramatically changing his food intake, he lost several kilograms. He began to feel much better within himself as he became stronger, fitter and more energised. This seemed to encourage a natural progression towards further dietary changes, implemented by Michael himself.

Gradually, over the next 12 months, Michael totally transformed his health, his body shape and, most importantly, his motivation and attitude towards his body. No pushing was necessary. In my experience, when someone is ready to take on such a challenge, they do it for the right reasons, complete with an abundance of motivation.

Today, three years later, Michael is a very successful fitness instructor – and boy, does he look awesome! He is able to maintain a balanced, sensible eating regimen (including the odd glass of wine and social dinner) using the principles of *Fat or Fiction*. His body fat is now a stable 13 per cent!

QUESTION   *But I don't want to go to the gym! Do I have to?*

ANSWER   No, you don't have to. It is certainly not compulsory in order to achieve the benefits of resistance training or cardiovascular conditioning. As previously mentioned, if you are a beginner, you may have to seek professional advice, even if it is just to get you started on the right track. Many personal trainers will be willing to come to your home and establish the most appropriate regimen for you to follow in privacy and comfort. It's quite amazing how little equipment you need to develop a very effective program.

Again, depending on your level of fitness and general physical capacity, you may decide to invest in a skipping rope, a 'Swiss ball', a medicine ball, some light dumbbells, an ab-roller, an exercise floor mat, a speed ball, a punching bag or an adjustable step. Your options are many and relatively inexpensive. With a bit of guidance and knowledge, you can even use bits and pieces from around the house (e.g. chairs or benches for doing push-ups and other 'body-weight'-related exercises, including abdominal crunches, squats and lunges). Obviously, a fully equipped gymnasium is the ideal place to put your body through its paces. Everyone must choose the method that is best for them, taking into account how much time they have available and any other commitments. Exercise programs can be undertaken at home very effectively. However, I do recommend that beginners seek professional guidance to avoid injuries.

WHAT OTHER FACTORS ALTER THE AMOUNT OF ENERGY YOU BURN?

The total energy you burn over any given 24-hour period is influenced by:

• your basal metabolic rate (BMR), which relates directly to your body composition
• physical activity (all movement)
• energy intake (size and composition of meals)
• thermogenesis (explained later in this chapter)
• age and sex
• growth
• pregnancy and breastfeeding
• hormonal influences
• genetic factors.

How do I calculate my LBW and BMR?

Once you have had your body composition analysed, calculate your LBW using the example on page 31 then use the chart below to estimate your BMR.

CALCULATING YOUR BMR

LBW	BMR		LBW	BMR	
KG	CALS	KJ	KG	CALS	KJ
35	1090	4556	65	2025	8465
36	1121	4686	66	2056	8594
37	1152	4815	67	2087	8724
38	1184	4949	68	2118	8853
39	1215	5079	69	2149	8983
40	1246	5208	70	2180	9112
41	1277	5338	71	2212	9246
42	1308	5467	72	2243	9376
43	1339	5597	73	2274	9505
44	1371	5731	74	2305	9635
45	1402	5860	75	2336	9764
46	1433	5990	76	2367	9894
47	1464	6119	77	2399	10028
48	1495	6249	78	2430	10157
49	1526	6379	79	2461	10287
50	1557	6508	80	2492	10416
51	1589	6642	81	2523	10546
52	1620	6772	82	2554	10676
53	1651	6901	83	2585	10805
54	1682	7031	84	2617	10939
55	1713	7160	85	2648	11069
56	1744	7290	86	2679	11198
57	1775	7419	87	2710	11328
58	1807	7553	88	2741	11457
59	1838	7683	89	2772	11587
60	1869	7812	90	2804	11721
61	1900	7942	91	2835	11850
62	1931	8072	92	2866	11980
63	1962	8201	93	2897	12167
64	1944	8126	94	2928	12298

Example

If 'Jim's' weight on the scales is 89 kg and his body-fat percentage is 20, his body-fat weight is 17.8 kg; therefore, his lean weight is the remaining 71.2 kg. Using the chart on page 30, we can calculate Jim's BMR as being approximately 2212 calories, or 9246 kj, per day.

QUESTION *Is it better to increase my physical activity or cut calories?*

ANSWER Commonly, the largest user of the energy you burn is your BMR, while physical activity is second on the list. Obviously, an increase in activity is a far more desirable way to lose weight than dramatically cutting your food consumption. Increased activity has many health benefits, and allows you to eat more, which in turn makes it easier for you to get sufficient nutrients for optimum health. A sedentary person is likely to have a considerably lower level of lean tissue and more body fat than an active one. The difference in calorie requirements is due to both a pattern of inactivity and the unfavourable body composition that results from this pattern.

QUESTION *How does eating affect my BMR?*

ANSWER Your metabolic rate actually increases after eating. The rise is determined by the quantity and composition of the meal and burns approximately 5 to 10 per cent of the calories consumed. The rate will peak approximately one hour after eating and return to normal four hours later. This is commonly known as the *thermic* effect of food. Obviously, increasing your thermic response doesn't give you an excuse to eat all day long.

QUESTION *Thermo-what?*

ANSWER In most regions of Australia, the temperature of our living environment is within a comfortable range. Even in more extreme conditions, many still have the luxury of airconditioning and heating. If we spend prolonged periods of time in extreme hot or cold temperatures, our energy requirements do change. The energy burned in temperatures below 14°C is around 5 per cent higher than would be burned if we were in a more comfortable environment. We all have a core temperature that our body likes to maintain. When we are exposed to cold temperatures, our body is stimulated to produce more energy (heat). This is why we shiver when cold. Shivering is an involuntary muscle contraction with the purpose of creating energy (heat) to keep us warm. Basically, if your body must work harder to maintain your core temperature (either by heating or cooling), you will have an increased requirement for energy. This is known as thermogenesis. For most of us, environmental change isn't great enough to warrant changing our calorie intake. The only significant effect climate has on energy expenditure is probably in the increases and decreases in our activity patterns. When an increase in temperature is triggered by ill health, our BMR can increase by approximately 10 per cent for every 0.6°C rise. Energy expenditure also increases in response to surgery or trauma.

QUESTION *Does energy requirement vary much between males and females?*
ANSWER Most height and weight charts are divided into male and female for the purpose of varying calorie requirements. One of the main reasons that this distinction is made is the obvious difference in the body composition of men and women. So the answer is yes, typically women will have less muscle and more fat. Lucky us!

I haven't made a lot of reference to men and women individually because most of the information I provide is based primarily on body composition anyway. Obviously men's and women's hormone levels are quite different, but again, the main effect these hormones have on your energy requirement is to create different body compositions for men and women.

What does age have to do with it?

Age is really only a relevant factor when there is a significant deterioration of lean tissue. As we age, many of us become less active and therefore burn fewer calories and have a slower metabolic rate. The trick is to stay active; if you do this, you will retain a desirable amount of lean tissue. Slow down, and your body will too – at any age. Statistically, an average adult's lean mass will decline by around 2 to 3 per cent per decade. Your BMR will decline proportionately.

Does growth influence the amount of energy I burn?

During phases of growth, energy is needed at a rate of approximately 5 calories per gram of growth tissue gained. Growth occurs, obviously, in childhood and adolescence but can also happen in adults as a result of exercise or even recovery from illness or injury. Apart from during the very early years of life, growth accounts for only a small amount (approximately 1 per cent) of the energy our bodies use.

Do I need to modify my calorie intake during pregnancy?

Most of us know that both pregnancy and breastfeeding increase our requirement for calories. This increase is obviously to accommodate added maternal tissues and growth of the foetus and placenta. However, I'm not convinced that we need to eat for two, because this is often interpreted as a need to eat enough food for two grown adults, from the very moment of conception.

Adequate weight gain during pregnancy, including some fat storage, is considered essential for supporting a healthy child. The chart on page 34 provides estimates of the increases in energy requirements during each stage of pregnancy and breastfeeding.

These figures are based on the assumption that you begin at an average weight for your height and maintain a 'normal range' of weight gain throughout the pregnancy (approximately 11 to 15 kg in total).

During the first six months of breastfeeding, you will produce an average of 750 ml of milk a day. This decreases to approximately 600 ml per day in the second six months. Breastfeeding will use approximately 85 calories for every 100 ml of milk produced. The extra calorie intake suggested, together with the stores of maternal fat, should meet your energy requirements.

CALORIES REQUIRED FOR PREGNANCY AND BREASTFEEDING

ACTIVITY	EXTRA CALORIES REQUIRED
PREGNANCY	
1st trimester	usually none
2nd trimester	approximately 300 per day
3rd trimester	approximately 300 per day
BREASTFEEDING	
1st six months	approximately 500 per day
2nd six months	approximately 500 per day

QUESTION   *What role do my genes and hormones play?*

ANSWER   There is at least another book in this subject alone. There are so many factors involved in genetics and hormonal influences. Some of us may encounter more genetic obstacles than others. Whether this is due to external circumstances or is genuinely influenced by our inherited make-up, it shouldn't prevent us from achieving our goals. However, if you find it all a bigger challenge than most people, the reward will be that much greater when you succeed.

QUESTION *I don't have time to exercise and I don't give fitness much priority in my life. Can I just eat less food and get similar results?*

ANSWER It all comes back to body composition, once again. You simply cannot eat less food than your BMR dictates without risking malnutrition and all of its associated problems, including muscle deterioration, lowered metabolism, a weakened immune system, illness and disease.

If you don't wish to create an exercise routine, then just make sure you remain very active. You cannot successfully reduce your calories below the level your body requires to compensate for inactivity. Firstly, it would be very difficult and stressful to maintain long term. Secondly, even if you did manage to cope, the longer you maintained this level, the more deterioration would result from lack of nourishment. In the process, your metabolism would become so sluggish that it would be close to impossible for you to lose fat or keep it at bay! You only get *one* body. It's such a small commitment to respect and maintain it. If you fail to maintain this body, where will you live out the last years of your life?

4

chapterfour

OVERWEIGHT AND UNDERNOURISHED

Refined foods and 'empty' calories

Sugar presents itself in many forms, including sucrose (table sugar), fructose (fruit sugar), lactose (milk sugar) and dextrose (corn sugar). The body breaks all of these down to glucose. Glucose is an essential body sugar used by all cells, including brain cells. However, it is not essential as a pure substance in our food.

Honey, raw sugar, natural fruit sugars etc. may not be quite as processed, but they are still very easily overconsumed, and the overall effect is pretty much the same.

As for other refined carbohydrates, such as white flour: it is probably best used to make wallpaper glue and papier-mâché!

The average English-speaking Western population consumes approximately 57 kg of sugar per person per annum. This equates to approximately 156 grams, or 9 to 10 tablespoons, of sugar per person per day. When you take into account that the average 340-ml can of soft drink contains 11.25 teaspoons of sugar, this statistic remains astonishing yet believable. That's right, it's not a misprint: *11.25 teaspoons!* Can you even begin to imagine devouring this amount of sugar in one sitting?

Following are lists of sometimes hidden sources of refined sugars and other carbohydrates in everyday use:

beverages and snacks soft drinks, cordials, commercial juices, yoghurt drinks, flavoured milks, some soy milks, iced tea, iced coffee, flavoured mineral water, cocktails, energy/sports drinks, many 'protein' drinks, milkshakes, low-fat/light yoghurts, ice-creams and dairy desserts, meal-replacement/diet drinks and snack foods, muesli and 'health' bars, coffee substitutes, 'healthy/low-fat' cakes, biscuits, crispbreads and muffins
condiments salad dressings, ketchup, mayonnaise etc.
flour products pasta, breads, crackers, pastries, cakes, muffins, biscuits, crispbreads.

SUGAR . . . NOT SO SWEET

It's always *fat* being portrayed as the villain, but you may find the following information quite astonishing.

Sugar depletes your body of B-complex vitamins and various minerals, thereby potentially increasing nervous tension, anxiety and irritability. Overconsumption can intensify fatigue by causing vasoconstriction (constriction of blood vessels). Numerous other health problems can be created or exacerbated. These include obesity, blood-sugar imbalances, dental decay, heart disease (elevated triglycerides or blood fats), arthritis (high uric acid – gout), hyperactivity, immunosuppression (decreased white blood cells) and diabetes. Sugar provides empty calories and potentially takes years off your life. Our immune system protects us from the invasion of viruses, bacteria, parasites, fungi, toxins, pollutants and even cancer. Recent studies suggest that sugar consumption can suppress the activity of white blood cells (neutrophils) by up to 50 per cent thirty minutes after ingestion and this immune-system suppression can last for up to six hours! This information is particularly disturbing when you consider what hospitals often feed patients.

Whether you consider refined sugar to be poison or you're a dedicated chocoholic, the most effective way to avoid the negative side effects of refined carbohydrates is to avoid consuming them. For ultimate blood-sugar control, combine unrefined carbohydrates with protein and essential fats.

The Centre for Science in the Public Interest, Washington DC, suggests that reducing sugar in soft drinks by one-tenth would reduce America's annual sucrose consumption by 480 million pounds!

case study sonya

In hindsight, Sonya would agree that, at twenty-seven years old, she was in a pretty bad state when we met in December 1999. At this time, we estimated her weight to have tipped the scales at around 180 kg. However, I was unable to get an accurate measure until we found some custom-made scales. It was quite a lot of excess weight for anyone to carry but especially for Sonya, who was only 163 cm tall. She had been given a copy of my first book, *Fat or Fiction*, by a concerned brother-in-law. She readily admits that her first thought was, 'Not another damned diet book.' However, she has confessed that after skimming through the first few pages she was so intrigued that she couldn't put it down.

Sonya decided to contact me for further advice. She planned to marry her long-time fiancé, Tony, in October 2000.

This allowed us only ten months to complete the daunting task of shedding those excess kilos. When I met Sonya, I knew immediately that she was ready to do this. All she needed was a little bit of direction and confidence. After all, she had amazing support from Tony, whose main concern was Sonya's health, which he had watched deteriorate over the past seven years.

We rearranged a multitude of things in Sonya's lifestyle, totally altering her food intake and gradually increasing her daily activity. Together, we set a goal to get Sonya's weight down to under 100 kg in time for her wedding day. By the time we managed to find suitable scales, Sonya weighed in at 159 kg. This meant that we had to aim for her to lose 60 kg in forty-four weeks – quite a task when you consider that she was attempting to shed the *total weight* of an average-sized woman.

In the first few weeks, Sonya found a five-minute walk difficult to complete without unbearable back pain. After a few months, she took it upon herself to join her local health club, where I set her a program consisting of cardiovascular exercise and weight training. She was hooked! Within weeks, she was walking on that treadmill as fast as her legs would carry her – sometimes for over an hour. This was a far cry from the girl hobbling around in a crippled state after a five-minute stroll.

With every passing week, Sonya's weight steadily declined. Throughout the entire pre-wedding schedule, her weight loss averaged approximately 1.5 kg per week. This sensible rate of weight loss allowed Sonya to consume a more-than-adequate quantity of all the essential nutrients. Most importantly, she didn't have to starve herself. At the time of writing this book, Sonya had lost a staggering 60 kg and was still going strong.

I am completely convinced that Sonya is now so accustomed to her new eating and exercise regimen that she will never look back. She has the sound knowledge necessary to maintain and manipulate her weight and remain in a healthy weight range for the rest of her life. She has mentioned on many occasions how she is surprised that it is all so easy, once you know how. I have no doubt that in years to come Sonya will impart her new-found knowledge and experience to others in similar situations.

Sonya Tanevska has excelled. I commend her for her relentless determination and willpower. We all know what it is like to motivate ourselves to lose 5 or 10 kg. But losing half your body weight is just mind-boggling. Wow! It just goes to show: where there's a will, there's a way.

Oh and by the way, she made a stunning bride.

ESTION *I understand the concept of consuming adequate nutrients. However, I find the whole subject very complicated. How do I keep track of what to eat and whether I need to take supplements?*

ANSWER You're right, it can be tricky. That is why I have been inspired to write this book for you. My intention is to give you all the answers that I possibly can, tailoring them to your individual requirements as much as possible. To achieve this, I have structured everything to correspond with your lean body weight (LBW), so all you need to do is have your body composition measured. Once you have this information, you will be able to use the calculations I have made to estimate your calorie requirements. Using my seven-day menu planner will ensure you maintain optimum nutritional balance. Sure, everyone is quite different, and with these variations comes a wide range of demand for nourishment. This is why you must learn to listen to the demands your body makes. Your body may require different quantities of vitamins and minerals at different stages of your life. If you are under a great deal of stress, are taking antibiotics or are recovering from surgery or illness, your requirements will be far greater than if you are relaxed and well. There are a couple of ways to address this.

• Eat a balanced diet (as suggested in the menu planner) and find yourself a multivitamin-and-mineral tablet to 'cover' yourself. This will contain a broad range of vitamins and minerals in relatively small quantities – enough to fill the gaps in most cases.
• If you feel that you put your body under a lot of stress (emotionally or physically), you may opt to seek professional advice from a naturopath or other health-care professional qualified to prescribe an individualised, appropriate supplement regimen for you. This may need to be revised and updated on a regular basis. Quite often, you can pick up a magazine and see an article about the benefits of a certain vitamin or mineral for a specific ailment. As beneficial as it may be, you must be aware that you should never just take one vitamin or mineral on its own without seeking advice first. For instance, many of the B-group vitamins need to be kept in balance with one another. B6 may be great for alleviating premenstrual tension and water retention in many cases, but you should always take the other B vitamins (B complex) in harmony. It can be detrimental to disturb the delicate balance required for optimum health. For this reason, I always recommend you take a multivitamin-and-mineral tablet containing vitamins and minerals in the appropriate ratios unless professionally advised otherwise.

QUESTION *If I'm carrying excess fat on my body, primarily as a result of overeating, surely my nutrition must be more than adequate . . . mustn't it?*

ANSWER Believe it or not, you are probably *starving* yourself. If you have been eating food that has caused excess fat storage, there is a good chance that it has been the *wrong* type of food and you have been *depriving* yourself of nourishment. By this, I mean you have probably been eating calorie-dense, nutrition-poor processed foods.

It is actually very difficult to eat too much *good* food. Think about it. Are you more likely to overindulge in steak and vegetables or desserts from your favourite restaurant? Yes . . . I thought so.

Often, very poor people are overweight because they live on inexpensive carbohydrates and are particularly unhealthy.

Nutrition aside for a moment, you can understand how easy it would be to miscalculate your food intake: if you were to compare similarly sized portions of 'real food' with highly processed foods, you might come up with very different energy values.

For example, which of the following two lunches would you choose?

OPTION 1	OPTION 2
ham, cheese and salad croissant with butter or margarine	large chef's salad of lean chicken, ham, egg, cheese and avocado dressed with balsamic vinegar
375 ml can of orange mineral water	375 ml can of 'diet' orange soft drink
1 caffelatte, 2 sugars	1 regular coffee with milk and approved sweetener
calories: 980	*calories: 350*

Both of the above meals would probably seem to be similar in quantity and make you feel equally satisfied, but what a difference in energy value! I don't think choosing option 2 would be considered by most people to be a big sacrifice. In fact, you'd probably enjoy it just as much as option 1, and feel a whole lot better for the rest of the day.

HAVE WE ALL
GONE MAD?

it's a dog's life

Next time you have the opportunity to read the recommended 'food pyramid' guide for your four-legged friend, you'll realise that it is actually a much healthier one than is recommended for humans. Essential fatty acids, bone-building calcium, and protein for repair and recovery actually get a mention in the dog's pyramid. I'm not suggesting that you start to eat puppy food for breakfast tomorrow morning. However, I will share a rather amusing story with you. It never ceases to amaze me that so many of us have such distorted food values. Quite recently, I was walking my dog at a local park. A woman and a young girl were walking their dog nearby. The child was eating from what appeared to be a packet of lollies. She tipped some into her hand and called to the dog, tempting him to investigate the contents. As the dog leapt up, the woman pushed the girl's hand away gasping, 'Don't feed the dog sweets! Don't you know it's bad for him? You should know better!' Ironically, the child apologised and, of course, ate the lollies herself. Obviously the woman had no problem with that – better, from her point of view, for the lollies to be in the child than the dog!

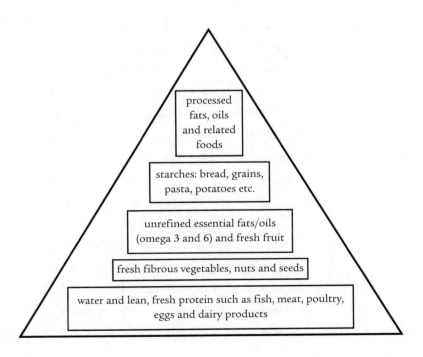

5

chapterfive

LET'S GO SHOPPING

Your new food pyramid: translating it into real food

In this chapter I will explain some terms you read on food labels. But first I will describe a food pyramid very different from the one we have worshipped for so long.

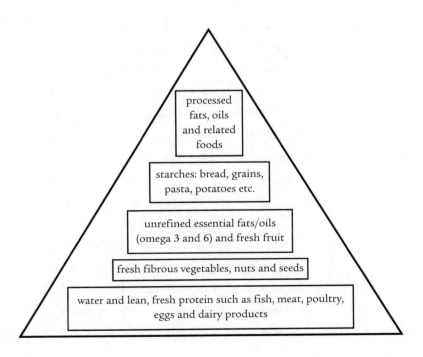

processed fats, oils and related foods

starches: bread, grains, pasta, potatoes etc.

unrefined essential fats/oils (omega 3 and 6) and fresh fruit

fresh fibrous vegetables, nuts and seeds

water and lean, fresh protein such as fish, meat, poultry, eggs and dairy products

Priority No. 1

WATER

MEAT   Fresh, lean fillet steak, rump steak, roast
                 (e.g. topside), porterhouse, T-bone, beef
                 mince, veal, pork and lamb

POULTRY   Skinless chicken, turkey, duck and quail

SEAFOOD   All varieties of fresh fish

                 Prawns, scallops, calamari, mussels, oysters,
                 crab, lobster, octopus etc.

                 Tinned fish such as salmon, tuna, sardines,
                 anchovies, mackerel and caviar (check labels
                 for additives and buy products packed in
                 water where possible)

                 Smoked fish such as salmon and cod (fresh
                 is preferred)

EGGS   Large-sized eggs (61 grams) are used in most
                 recipe calculations in this book

DAIRY PRODUCTS   Milk (limited due to lactose content)

                 Cheeses (reduced fat or full cream specified
                 in menu planner) such as cheddar, edam,
                 mozzarella, parmesan, brie, camembert,
                 gouda, fetta, cottage (plain), ricotta, cream
                 cheese

                 Yoghurt (reduced fat or full cream specified
                 in menu planner) – read labels and avoid
                 items containing added sugar, including
                 honey, dextrose, fructose and sucrose;
                 choose Diet Lite or 'natural' varieties – the
                 fewer additives the better (preferred brands
                 will contain less than 15 grams of

carbohydrate per 200 grams)
Butter (not butter substitutes), cream
Whey protein concentrate (choose a brand
with no added sugars) – a wide selection of
protein powders is available in your local
health-food shop

The protein foods listed above are actively associated with many essential functions within the body. Protein is responsible for forming enzymes, haemoglobin to transport oxygen in the blood, and antibodies to keep our immune system strong and healthy. We need a constant supply of amino acids to build and repair our body tissues. Hair, nails and all living cells are always growing or requiring replacement. Protein is responsible for all these functions. Red blood cells last about a month, as do skin cells, while cells that line our intestinal tract are replaced twice every week. During times of illness, stress or surgery, we require even more protein to regenerate vital cells and tissues.

Priority No. 2

VEGETABLES   Fresh salad greens (e.g. lettuce), tomatoes
                       (technically fruit), cucumbers, capsicums (all
                       colours), cauliflower, brussels sprouts, green
                       beans, carrots, cabbage, onions, spring
                       onions, leeks, pumpkin, spinach, eggplant,
                       mushrooms, snow peas, bok choy, squash,
                       zucchini, broccoli, asparagus, artichokes,
                       beetroot, celery, garlic etc.; frozen 'plain'
                       vegetables may be used, but check labels to
                       ensure the absence of unnecessary

additives – 'fresh' is always preferred to
tinned, dried or sun-dried

NUTS AND SEEDS   Raw, not roasted, including almonds,
cashews, hazelnuts, macadamias, pecans and
walnuts

Nut pastes with no additives or sugar, such
as almond paste

Sesame seeds, pumpkin seeds, sunflower
seeds, linseeds

Seed pastes with no additives or sugar, such
as tahini (sesame paste)

Psyllium husks

This food group provides us with the majority of our fibre,
essential fats and anti-oxidants. A wide variety of these foods will
help to ensure a good balance of nourishment, as well as that all-
important feeling of satiety.

Priority No. 3

OILS   Unrefined/cold-pressed oils (omega 3 and
omega 6): olive oil or 'high oleic'
sunflower/safflower oils for cooking;
flaxseed oil or Omega Balance combination
oil (refrigerated at most health-food shops)
as salad oil

FRUIT   Seasonal fresh fruit is always preferable; if
purchasing packaged fruit, always ensure it is
packaged in its natural juice, with no added
sugars; frozen fruit is okay as long as it is free
of additives; no dried fruit should be

consumed; apples, melons, strawberries, raspberries, blackberries, passionfruit, mandarins, avocado, kiwifruit, pineapple, grapefruit, apricots, peaches, lemons, limes, nectarines, oranges etc.

I can't stress enough the importance of *unrefined oils*. Whether they are derived from a plant or from oily fish, they must be unspoilt. Essential fats assist in the maintenance of a healthy cardiovascular system, the reduction of inflammatory conditions and the prevention of a variety of common health problems. .

A daily intake of fresh fruit provides us with fibre, vitamins, minerals and essential anti-oxidants. Nature has perfectly created a combination of essential nutrients in an easy-to-eat and tasty food.

Priority No. 4

GRAINS, STARCHY VEGETABLES, RICE, CEREAL ETC.	Preferred cereal grains are rolled oats, oat bran, wheat bran and wheat germ; mountain bread and high-fibre, whole-grain breads; all high-starch/high-carbohydrate vegetables, including potatoes, corn and sweet potatoes; unpolished brown rice, which is the highest-fibre, least-processed variety

The same basic rules apply here: *unprocessed and unrefined*. If it's an unrecognisable powder, or if it's presented in a pretty, colourful box boasting a list of ingredients a mile long, don't eat it! Try your local health-food shop or organic grocer. You'll probably find a more appealing variety.

'Priority' No. 5

PROCESSED FATS, OILS AND RELATED FOOD PRODUCTS	This range of 'so-called food' should be avoided completely, but I have listed the best of a bad bunch: processed/ manufactured deli meats, including ham, bacon, salami, pastrami, sausages, frankfurters and chicken loaf can be consumed occasionally

Margarines and spreads, refined vegetable oils, deep-fried foods, bakery products (cakes etc.), chocolate, ice-cream, pies, sausage rolls, tinned ham, spring rolls, dim sims, hot dogs, most packaged meals, fried rice and tinned pasta should always be avoided.

My best advice is that you walk away from these 'food imitations'. They are probably all full of harmful trans-fatty acids. If you eat them there will only be one positive side – when you do die an early death, at least your corpse will be well preserved.

To reiterate, then: all adults should consume a minimum of 1.5 litres of pure water daily and eat adequate lean, fresh protein foods, including fish, several times per week; two of your daily meals should include a variety of colourful vegetables; raw nuts and seeds (not roasted) are a nutritious and very convenient snack; unrefined essential oils (such as omega 3 and omega 6) are of utmost importance in a healthy, balanced diet – adults require at least 1 tablespoon of these oils daily; you should also eat a few pieces of fresh fruit daily, limit consumption of heavy starches, such as bread, potatoes and pasta, eliminate all sources of highly processed saturated (animal) and unsaturated (plant) fats and oils and eliminate as many refined, 'empty' foods as possible, including sugar, white flour, packaged and processed food products, chemicals and additives.

case study stephen

Although losing body fat wasn't Stephen's first priority, he made the decision to change his dietary habits. He had studied my principles and recognised that he could probably do many things to improve his general wellbeing. The major stumbling block he encountered was the supermarket! Not unlike most of us, Stephen was a creature of habit. His usual routine included a 10-minute whiz around the supermarket aisles that he could have accomplished blindfolded. He soon discovered that adding different food and ingredients to his shopping list meant he had to pick up items and read the labels – what a time-consuming pain, right? Suddenly, he found his food-shopping expeditions were consuming almost 40 minutes of his time. But after two weeks Stephen had it down pat. It had simply been a challenge to change his long-time habits. As Stephen now agrees, it really is no more difficult to shop this way, just a bit different.

An added bonus of eliminating many of his usual processed food choices was that Stephen's grocery bill was reduced dramatically. As he now realises, once you become familiar with your new-found products, you're back to your 10-minute 'whiz' in no time.

QUESTION *What about those commercial food products that claim to be fortified with added nutrients?*

ANSWER The bottom line is, if something has had to have nutrients put back into it, it may also, at some stage, have had them removed. This makes it a pretty undesirable 'food substitute' in my view. The other problem lies in the imbalance of nutrients. Each and every whole food has a very intricate balance of nutrients. How could we even hope, let alone be sure, that any laboratory would be capable of achieving the same balance? Sure, manufacturers may fortify a cereal or bread with fibre and iron, but the original product has generally been so severely processed initially that much of its natural goodness has gone. It is not worthy of passing your lips, really. Many more nutrients would have been destroyed than the two or three being replaced, leaving you with a nutritionally unbalanced food product far different from the one nature intended.

WHAT ARE YOU *REALLY* EATING?

The intention of food preservation is to prevent spoilage and thereby avoid food poisoning and prolong products' shelf life. There are many preserving methods, some with potentially detrimental health effects. The following list briefly explains what you are eating.

Canning

You only need walk down a supermarket aisle to see the thousands of products available in cans – everything from fruit and vegetables to chocolate ants. The process of canning can destroy potassium and vitamins A, B1 and C, depending on the food in question. Nutrition values aside, improperly processed meats are prone to botulin contamination. Cans that are distorted, swollen or dented can harbour poisonous substances. If tin cans do not have an interior coating, an undesirable amount of tin can leach into the food, which we then consume.

Freezing

The freezing of foods requires storage at temperatures below freezing point (usually at minus 18°C), and this can affect certain nutrients, including folic acid and vitamins B5, C and E. If commercially frozen foods are not handled and transported properly and defrost then refreeze as a result, they may harbour substances that can cause food poisoning. Be wary of food containing ice crystals or in swollen packaging.

Partial Hydrogenation

Whoever invented this process should be *fully* hydrogenated. This common industrial process uses hydrogen gas at high temperatures to change unsaturated fatty acids (UFAs), or plant oils, into mutated substances to simplify packaging and marketing.

Partial hydrogenation improves the colour of oil. It transforms liquid oils into solid 'user-friendly' but deformed products. It also converts UFAs into chemically modified (i.e. artificial) fats that are less susceptible to free-radical damage – in other words, they last longer on the shelf and manufacturers make more *dosh*!

So what's wrong with processing oils in this way? It transforms naturally occurring fats into highly toxic trans-fatty acids (TFAs). It results in many unnatural and some unknown by-products called altered fats. Although not thoroughly researched to date, I can't even begin to imagine their cumulative toxic effects. Partial hydrogenation is a part of the manufacturing process of most margarine and therefore of its related products.

Pasteurisation

This process is most commonly applied to milk and other dairy products. It involves the mild heating of a product, followed by immediate cooling. Its purpose is to destroy many forms of harmful bacteria that may be present in food. On the down side, it destroys 10 to 20 per cent of vitamins B1 and C in food. It also destroys the enzymes that contribute to the therapeutic benefits of miso (a soya product).

Smoking

This process is commonly used to cure or flavour food. The problem lies in the presence of a chemical known as benzpyrene. It is formed as a result of the heat applied in food processing and has been proved to cause cancer in humans. Other sources of this chemical are overheated frying oils and charred meats.

Ionising Electromagnetic Radiation

They do this to food? You bet they do!

This is a pretty controversial method of food preservation involving gamma rays. Aside from the destruction of countless vitamins and enzymes naturally present in our food, it can open a whole new can of worms.

• It can make food more susceptible to fungi.

• Potatoes contaminated by solanine (which is toxic) will not turn green if they have been irradiated. As a result, people could unwittingly consume this toxin.

• Consumption of irradiated food is suspected of increasing the risk of some forms of cancer.

• Irradiation can diminish or destroy vitamins A, C, E, K, B1, B2, B3, B6, B12 and carotene.

Some of the foods that are most commonly irradiated are meat and fish (to preserve them), citrus fruit (to prevent insect infestation), mangoes (to delay ripening), and onions and potatoes (to inhibit sprouting).

Pickling

Food is pickled using acids, such as vinegar or salt brine. Too much of these foods (particularly pickled vegetables) may increase the risk of oesophageal and stomach cancer. Everything in moderation.

Refrigeration

Although we all use refrigeration without a second thought, it may be worth checking your refrigerator to ensure it is keeping everything at the appropriate temperature. Use a refrigerator thermometer to check this. Obviously, it is an effective way to preserve our food and inhibit the formation of many harmful bacteria. Never keep food for too long in the fridge and always discard food when the use-by date expires. If in doubt, throw it out.

Homogenisation

Milk is forced through small holes at high pressure to emulsify the fats and prevent the cream from separating.

Cooking Methods

On the positive side, cooking can destroy certain bacteria and food toxins, as well as improve the digestibility of meat and vegetables.

On the negative side, heat can destroy many vitamins and nutrients that are naturally present in our food. The application of heat of more than 160°C also destroys many beneficial fats and can convert essential fats into TFAs, which have been proved to be detrimental to health.

Heat also destroys choline, folic acid and vitamins B1, B2, B6 and B12.

Following are a few of the basic rules of healthy cooking:

• Never overcook or char food.

• Don't boil vegetables or many water-soluble vitamins will be poured down the sink with the water they were cooked in. Steam, microwave, lightly stir-fry or oven bake. When it comes to vegetable preparation, aim for 'crunchy', not 'soggy'.

• Don't deep fry or use overheated cooking oils. Never, ever, ever reuse cooking oils. Use nonstick cookware to reduce the need for excess oil.

Synthetic Preservatives

Many processed meats contain a veritable cocktail of preservatives and additives. You will find some of the most detrimental synthetic preservatives in abundance in our beloved ham. These preservatives are known as nitrites. Nitrites can combine with amino acids in the stomach to form nitrosamines, which are extremely potent carcinogens capable of causing many forms of cancer. Vitamins C and E, strawberries, garlic and tea can inhibit this conversion. However, this doesn't mean that I recommend eating the 'poison' just because you have access to the 'antidote'. Nitrites are being phased out of many foods today because of their toxicity.

Leavening Agents/Baking Powder

This group of food additives produces bubbles of gas in dough or batter to facilitate rising. Toxic minerals such as aluminium are often used in these additives. You may be thinking, 'Well, I'm safe because I don't really use baking powders in my cooking.' Think again. How many commercially prepared products do you actually consume on a daily basis that contain baking powder? Read the labels and think about it.

Colouring

One of the most common colouring agents known to have adverse effects on health is tartrazine. Also known by numerous other names and numbers, it is basically yellow food colouring. In sensitive people, it may cause hives as well as induce asthma and other allergic reactions.

Genetically Modified Foods, or 'Frankenfood'

Technology today is amazing. Can you believe that it is now possible to genetically engineer our food? It's quite a controversial subject. If you don't really know what it's all about, then I suggest you read this section, because you probably have a fridge full of the stuff.

DNA is the substance that carries our unique genetic information, or our genes. It's like a blueprint for every component of every living thing, from humans and plants to bacteria and viruses. As you are probably aware, our genes determine an array of individual traits, such as the colour of our hair and skin. There are 100 000 known genes in mammals, and there is no doubt that every living thing has some genetic traits that are desirable and some that are not.

Technology has advanced to a stage where the genetic material from different species can be spliced together. This allows technologists the freedom to create foods with the characteristics of another living species. It is the movement between species that is of the greatest concern. Hence, 'Frankenfood'. Why would anyone want to do this?

In agriculture, crops can be spliced with genes to make them resistant to herbicides and chemicals. For the farmers, this is revolutionary stuff. Now they can spray their crops with a greater variety of chemicals, killing weeds and parasites, allowing a far more successful harvest. Unfortunately, we get to eat the chemical-drenched food.

There have been many instances of cross-species genetic engineering involving everyday foods. What about fish genes being spliced into tomatoes to reduce freezer damage – hard to believe but true. At present, we have no way of distinguishing between modified foods and the natural ones. Many products will state that they are free of genetically modified organisms (GMOs), but many manufacturers of commercial products are probably unaware of the genetic modification of some ingredients they use. In a newspaper article that I read recently, a reporter had phoned a corn-chip manufacturer to ask if the company used GM corn. The answer? 'We don't know.' Apparently the manufacturer receives produce from four different suppliers and claims to have no way of knowing which corn is GM and which is not. We may now have the technology to break through nature's cross-species barrier, but at what cost?

Food intolerances and allergies may also be an issue with GM foods. As GM foods don't presently have to be identified as such on food labels in all countries, allergic reactions may be difficult for consumers to avoid. A person with a known allergy to fish isn't in his or her wildest dreams going to expect an adverse reaction to a tomato, but this is exactly what can happen. One horrific incident resulting from meddling with nature is 'mad cow disease'. Researchers believe that this epidemic may have resulted from feeding cows a meal consisting of the ground-up remains of dead cattle. Genetically modifying food could enable unnatural foods to be introduced into our own food supply.

It is almost impossible to avoid consuming GM foods. Many

informed manufacturers are now stating the absence of these foods in their product, but how many are saying nothing? Where possible, select organic fresh foods, and when purchasing products derived from crops such as soy, ensure that they are clearly labelled 'GMO free'.

In early 1999, the Australia New Zealand Food Authority gave health and safety approval for the testing of the first two genetically modified food products, under a new set of Australian rules. You might be surprised to discover that both of those foods were already on the supermarket shelves. The Australia New Zealand Food Standards Council has approved new food standards to ensure the safety of GM foods. This regulation has been enforced since May 1999. After many years of debate, Australian federal and state ministers have agreed that, as of July 2001, all food products containing GMOs must be labelled, which will make ours the most rigid standard in the world to date. The exceptions to this ruling are restaurant and take-away meals, highly refined sugars and starches and processing agents and additives with GM material in the final product. At present, up to 65 per cent of food on Australian supermarket shelves has GM content.

The major sources of GM ingredients to date are US imported soy and Australian-grown cotton. Cottonseed oil from that cotton goes into such products as margarine. What other GM products have been or are being produced or trialled in Australia? Lupins, canola, salmonella and bovine herpes virus vaccines, potatoes, tomatoes, carnations, cotton and sugar cane.

HAVE WE ALL
GONE MAD?

the perfect garnish

Have you ever noticed that vegetables are becoming more of a garnish than part of the meal? I'm harking back to the USA on this subject because, once again, people there seem to have this one down pat. And we all know that what happens in the USA usually happens here sooner or later. Now, call me old-fashioned, but I like to eat my vegetables as part of my meal rather than look at them as a colourful plate decoration! Just recently, while on that trip to the USA, I was in a restaurant for dinner when I was presented with a huge dinner plate. I ordered a fillet steak, no sauce, and the chef's vegetables du jour. In the centre of my plate was a lovely piece of steak, and meticulously arranged around the edges were three finely grated strips of orange (carrot, I presume), a carefully twisted slice of green (perhaps a bean?), and an almost triangular slice of yellow (now I'm almost positive this was button squash). Sure, it looked like a work of art, but where was my dinner?

Many restaurants these days seem to be serving rather large plates full of things like rice, every style of potato, or pasta. But what has happened to the vegetables? I have found that, particularly in America, everything seems to be about getting the most (quantity-wise) for your money. Everywhere you turn you see a sign saying, 'All you can eat for only $5.95.' The buffets are unbelievable. At a recent hotel breakfast buffet, I was amazed by the sheer volume of food people were consuming just because it didn't cost any more to eat twice as much. I'm sure they would have made themselves physically ill, all before nine o'clock in the morning. The waiters were so accustomed to this that if they attempted to put bread on the table and we declined it, they would splutter, 'But it's complimentary!' If you still didn't want it, they would look at you as if you were mad.

6

chaptersix

THE PROBLEM WITH DIETS

It's not your fault

What could possibly be wrong with eating low fat? After all, it's the healthy thing to do, right? After reading this chapter, you can decide for yourself.

LOW-FAT DIETS

Following are some negative aspects of eating the low-fat way.

• Lack of fat often renders food quite unpalatable, causing food manufacturers to plump up our fat-depleted food with all sorts of thickeners and sweeteners. This is not an ideal trade-off.

• Fat-reduced foods will leave you feeling hungry all day, generating low-grade irritability. It is most certainly very stressful to be hungry. In this day and age, I think you would agree that most of us don't need added stress.

• For the above two reasons, you will most likely increase your consumption of carbohydrates both to satisfy your hunger and, inadvertently, by consuming the unseen additives in many low-fat products. Many of these additional carbohydrates will be of the refined variety – calorie rich and nutrition poor.

• This unsatisfying way of eating is very difficult to maintain. Quite recently, a British study revealed that individuals on a low-fat diet were more likely to be inconsistent in their eating habits than those consuming a moderate amount of desirable fats.

• Inadequate fats in the diet will hinder your ability to absorb fat-soluble vitamins. Even if these vitamins are taken in supplement form, they cannot be effectively utilised by your body in the absence of fat. Many of these vitamins are anti-oxidants, which protect your body from numerous degenerative processes.

• Without adequate dietary fat, your body may be stimulated to manufacture more cholesterol. There is a lot more to that old cholesterol theory of eating less dietary fats than many people realise. Unfortunately, too many medical professionals are still preaching the incomplete theory by failing to distinguish between the good and bad sources of dietary fat.

Within the framework of clinical nutrition, a low-fat diet is theoretically unsound and generally ineffective.

HIGH-CARBOHYDRATE DIETS

The high-carbohydrate diet would have to be the most commonly prescribed way of eating. It's based on that outdated and, frankly, wrong traditional food pyramid. I'm not discounting the fact that your body does need a certain amount of carbohydrate. However, the word carbohydrate is a very broad term describing an enormous food group. It is an umbrella category for many different foods. Sometimes, deciphering which foods belong to this group can be confusing. Whether the items are in the form of refined sugars, grains, cereals and flours, vegetables, fruit or the thousands of derivatives of these foods, they all go into the vast carbohydrate category. The more a food is processed, the less nutritional value and fibre it contains.

Many people believe that if they don't sprinkle sugar on their porridge or in their coffee, then they are safe from raging insulin. So many times I have heard people say, 'But I don't have sugar in anything!' What you may not realise is that all refined carbohydrates trigger the same response as pure sugar when ingested. Even when you eat savoury food such as pizza base, a rice cake or a slice of bread, your insulin response is sugar, sugar, sugar.

Carbs: we need them for energy, right? We're currently told by 'experts' worldwide to consume around 70 per cent of our daily calories in the form of carbohydrates. Let's say you're following a low-fat, low-calorie diet of around 1200 calories in an attempt to lose weight. Seventy per cent of those calories is equivalent to 840 calories, leaving just 360 calories for other foods. If only 15 per cent of this diet was fat, fats and carbohydrates would account for a whopping 85 per cent (1020 calories) of energy-based foods. What must we do with this energy to prevent it from being stored as body fat? Burn it! We are taught that if we feel low in energy we must need more carbohydrates, or sugars, as a pick-me-up. What we probably need are more calories, full stop. More specifically, we need nutritious calories from real food.

The value of bulk/fibre and essential nutrients is often overlooked, as is the rate at which sugars are released and absorbed by the blood. All carbohydrates are not created equal. The more processed carbohydrates are, the less nutrients and fibre are available and the quicker the sugars are released, creating a very unstable blood-sugar level. Low blood sugar (hypoglycaemia) may result, with symptoms ranging from headache, dizziness, nausea, sweets cravings and trembling to heart palpitations and insatiable hunger. It's far too easy to overeat processed carbohydrates. I am suggesting that you can eat virtually unlimited amounts of vegetables, along with sufficient fruit and other natural and unprocessed foods. You will soon discover that when fibre and bulk remain intact, it is almost impossible to overeat these foods, even when you try.

HIGH-PROTEIN DIETS

To me, the word 'high' in this context usually refers to 'more than adequate'. As long as many people are consuming far *less than adequate* quantities of protein, I don't feel it's necessary or beneficial to health to embrace a 'high-protein' diet. Many diets on the market today preach the high-protein, low-carbohydrate, high-fat philosophy. Their claims are often as extreme as their food choices. Sure, you can lose weight quite quickly on some of these plans. However, it is rarely sustainable for long periods and is not particularly good for your health.

Why would it be necessary to consume 'too much' of any nutrient, e.g. protein?

Usually to compensate for a lack of whatever food is being restricted. In the case of high-protein diets, it is generally carbohydrate that is restricted. Severely restricting carbohydrates can result in weight loss but has various side effects. Quite often, diets in which vegetables and fresh fruit are severely restricted lack fibre, anti-oxidants and countless other nutrients. I consider these essential components of any diet. Not only are you likely to regain the weight when willpower fails, but you may also find yourself left with many nutritional deficiencies and associated ailments.

One of the major drawbacks of the common low-carb,

high-protein weight-loss methods is that quite often they are not nutritionally balanced. They tend to focus on ratios of protein, carbohydrates and fats. In other words, the attitude is that as long as you consume protein and fats while severely restricting your carbohydrates, it doesn't really matter where these foods come from. These diets often recommend highly processed sources of protein and fat, regardless of their detrimental effect on your health. Critics of these diets argue that too much protein affects your kidney and liver function and that too much animal fat is bad for you. My main opposition to them is that they are terribly unbalanced. They lack many vital nutrients and usually consist of far too many processed fats. Whether or not these fats are derived from animals or vegetables is not as important as whether or not they have been transformed into toxic substances.

THE HYPE ABOUT BLOOD TYPE!

Now we're being told that our blood type determines what nutrition we require. It's kind-of like saying that if you have red hair you should eat fish, but if you have black hair it's crucial that you avoid red meat.

We now have quite a selection of diets to choose from. With such stiff competition, I suppose that from a marketing point of view they've decided to come up with something unique. Guess what? The marketing *did* work, regardless of the diet!

The basic premise is that our blood type can somehow determine what foods are best for our health. I must admit that I have a real problem getting my head around some of the claims made, and an even harder time finding research to back it up.

I had an amusing conversation with a friend who happens to be a doctor. He loves this whole blood-type concept. Why? I'm not sure. Perhaps he and the author both have blood type B: they get the best diet. The first time we discussed this topic, my friend said, 'I bet you're a type O, because you're so slim and active and you thrive on exercise!' I laughed at the suggestions, replying, 'So does that mean that fifteen years ago, when I was a fat couch potato, I had a different blood type?' I'm sure you can understand my sarcasm. As we all know, changing our blood type is physically impossible. However, changing our body type is certainly not. As someone who spends a large percentage of her waking hours studying nutrition-related research, I have yet to discover one paragraph of data to justify these claims. Dietary requirements should be based on a few factors (and I'm afraid that blood type isn't one of them). These factors are:

• goals/lifestyle
• nourishment required by an individual
• state of health at various stages of life
• the presence of illness, disease or medications
• whether nourishment is required for maintenance of a healthy body or for repair of an unwell one.

BUT IT ALL SOUNDS SO LOGICAL

I have been listening to a few audio books lately and I must say that it's not hard to understand how we can be drawn in by some of these gurus. With the universal desperation to lose weight come the opportunists who would recommend chewing your arms off to lose weight, if they could get away with it.

My advice is not to take everything you hear or read on the subject of dieting at face value. Require arguments to be logical and soundly based.

THE DELICATE SUBJECT OF EATING DISORDERS

I must admit that until I received a phone call one day thanking me for addressing the subject of eating disorders in *Fat or Fiction* I had actually decided to delete this section. Why? Because it is a very delicate subject and by no means my area of expertise. Deciding to include the section was something I agonised over for some time. However, I have a great deal of contact with women with varying degrees of eating problems and I feel extremely concerned about their plight. The number of our younger people being exposed to distorted body images and adopting extreme diets is increasing, and for this reason I feel compelled to comment on the subject once again.

I think that eating disorders are still quite a mystery, both to those who suffer from them and those who do not. Why on earth would a seemingly healthy person just choose not to eat? Or purge food after eating? It is obviously a very complex problem, involving both physical and psychological issues that I don't claim to be capable of addressing professionally. However, I'd like to share some personal observations with you.

Quite recently, I viewed yet another documentary about eating disorders. Four young girls suffering from anorexia nervosa were admitted for between fourteen and sixteen weeks to a local hospital specialising in eating disorders. Each of the girls seemed to know very little about food and nutrition. They were chronically ill and undernourished, most of them weighing under 40 kg. The treatment program involved feeding the girls a 'meal replacement' drink several times per day and weighing them on the scales every second day. Why do I find this disturbing? The treatment program didn't seem to address the subject of nutrition education, which might have helped them establish healthy eating habits. They were just being *fed*. Surely a sugar-filled drink is not exactly the nourishment needed. Sure, it will make you put weight on when you jump on the scales – but what sort of weight? Some may argue that it is better nourishment than they were feeding themselves, but in my view, force-feeding and fattening-up can't cure eating disorders. Food seemed to be perceived as punishment. If the girls didn't gain the weight expected by the doctor, they were punished by being fed more calories and were restrained from moving so they would conserve more energy. They were given no responsibility for their condition. I understand the view that it might be their lack of responsibility that got them into such a state to begin with. However, I actually don't see it this way. This disorder will quite often be the result of extreme self-control. The girls' desire is to refrain from eating and they have obviously done this very successfully. Perhaps a shift in the direction of that relentless focus is a more positive step to take? This didn't happen to them by accident: their weight loss was intentional! If these girls could achieve such an unhealthy, undernourished state, I believe that they could also achieve the opposite, given the appropriate direction and education.

I understand that when a person gets to the stage at which their health and even their survival are threatened by such an illness, drastic measures must be employed and enforced. However, I can't help thinking that there has to be a more positive treatment process – one that will encourage the patient to participate and become more independent. After all, we are talking about a daily personal function (feeding ourselves), not a thing that one can be forced to do for a lifetime, unless, of course, 24-hour surveillance can be provided.

The weight these girls were gaining was fat. Just imagine how terrifying this would be to someone for whom fat is the enemy. More emphasis could be placed on body composition than on a reading from bathroom scales. It seems to me that this current widely used method of treatment is reinforcing the sufferers' worst nightmare: the scales are being used to measure progress, regardless of what kind of weight is being gained (fat or lean). It seems to prove to the girls that being heavier means getting fatter. And they are right in their case, because the weight they are gaining *is* predominantly fat, partially because they move around so little while in hospital. Until they understand the difference between good weight and bad weight, they will probably continue to believe that they must remain light on the scales in order to keep the fat at bay.

I am aware that it can be unhealthy, mentally and physically, to focus so much on the way we look. However, in my brief experience with this subject, many sufferers of eating disorders appear to have quite obsessive personalities – are perfectionists, you might say. I don't think it is likely that the very essence of their personality would, or even should, change, but perhaps just a little bit of education could go a long way towards helping them achieve more promising results.

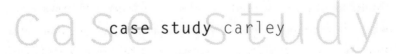

case study carley

Carley had spent the bulk of her forty-one years surrounded by ballet. The first time I heard her voice on the other end of a telephone, she sounded tired and frail. From her early teens, Carley had been battling with an eating disorder destructive enough to dominate her life. Though she was determined to pursue her career, the standard of perfection she set for herself was practically unachievable. With each

perceived *failure*, Carley appeared to slump further into a
deep depression, leading to self-punishing behaviour, usually in the form of starvation.

Many years after retiring from dance, she was still seeking advice from every diet-related publication she could get
her hands on. This is when Carley read *Fat or Fiction* and
decided to contact me for further advice. In her words, 'It
was as though somebody had turned the light on! Finally,
it began to make sense.' Many of the health problems she
had suffered were clearly a result of her starvation and
malnutrition.

I keep in contact with Carley and she is still going strong.
It has been quite an accomplishment for her to gain the confidence to eat, without the immense feeling of guilt. Carley
has now experienced the comfortable feeling of satiety one
gets from eating the *right* food. She has quite a long road
ahead, but at least she is travelling in the right direction.

QUESTION   *How can I be confident that this plan is different from all the others?*

ANSWER   Perhaps the only way to really find out is to try to experience the
results for yourself. If what you have been doing in the past is not
working for you, it is definitely time for a change. Mine is an unbi-
ased approach. In this book I have attempted to provide you with
the most personalised program possible in this form. I believe the
diet industry fails to provide tailored programs meeting the calorie requirements and nutritional needs of your individual body
composition. I can tell you that I have witnessed success hundreds
and hundred of times. Apart from a few excess kilos of fat, what
have you got to lose?

QUESTION *I've followed many different low-fat and low-calorie diets in the past and have lost weight. How can you say that they don't work when I have seen results for myself?*

ANSWER I think you've answered your own question. In my opinion, any diet that you have tried many times didn't work, unless you consider yo-yo weight loss and gain success. Weight fluctuation of any substantial degree can be detrimental to your health. If these diets were so difficult to maintain, there's a chance that they were either calorie deficient, nutritionally deficient or both.

The earlier chapters on body composition and yo-yo dieting explain why the weight keeps creeping back on and why these diets and results cannot be maintained.

One example of weight fluctuation is evident in one of my most recent clients, Sonya. You can read her story in the Case Study in Chapter 4.

HAVE WE ALL
GONE MAD?

surgery without success

Let me tell you a rather horrendous story of a desperate, medically bungled attempt at weight loss. After her first child, Judy gained close to 50 kg, bringing her total weight up to 110 kg. This was almost double the weight her tiny frame had once carried. Her doctor expressed concern at her high blood pressure. He suggested that if she lost weight, her blood pressure would return to normal. He suggested that she needed to lose the weight very quickly and that her best option was stomach stapling. All it would take was a small incision near her breastbone. The operation would reduce her appetite and her weight problem would be solved. Judy thought that this sounded quite simple, so she agreed.

To her horror, Judy ended up with a scar from her breastbone to her navel. Even though she was only able to consume liquids over the next few months she lost just over the 15 kg. Judy's weight was still hovering around 95 kg and her blood pressure remained unchanged. Her doctor now suggested that she should begin taking medication to lower her blood pressure, as it was a risk to her health. In response to Judy's depression and feelings of disappointment at her lack of success, her doctor prescribed antidepressant medication.

I met Judy ten years later, still on both prescribed drugs, still 95 kg and still desperately
unhappy and unhealthy. She was only able to eat soft,
mushy food as a result of her operation. She avoided
all vegetables and fruit, along with most 'real,
whole foods' due to the difficulty she had digesting
them. The easiest food for her to eat was sweet biscuits. She would even gag while eating an apple
unless she sat and chewed every bite for ten or fifteen minutes. Many fibrous foods would automatically
be regurgitated, much to her disgust. As a result of
her lack of nutritious food, her skin was dry and
cracked, and now - the last straw - her hair was
beginning to fall out. She approached her doctor for
a solution, but was told she couldn't have the operation reversed. Her stomach has been stapled, which
means that the staples have perforated the stomach
wall and cannot be removed. Even if they could be
removed, her stomach would now be twice the size it
used to be, having stretched to accommodate her present food consumption.

Judy's doctor offered to prescribe more medication
to assist in digestion, but finally Judy decided
she'd had enough. We are currently working on a diet
format, slowly increasing quantities of 'real foods'
to supply adequate nutrition while allowing her body
to shed some excess fat. Finally, Judy feels she has
control of her situation, but what an expensive, dan-
gerous and totally unnecessary lesson to learn!

7

chapterseven

BURN, BABY, BURN!

*How to influence your body to choose
stored body fat for fuel*

Overindulgence in refined carbohydrates can lead to hypoglycaemia, or low blood-sugar levels. Most of the time, you
don't need a fancy test to tell you whether this is a problem
you experience. You only need ask yourself how you feel after having eaten nothing for four hours, or after having eaten sugar.

INSULIN AND GLUCAGON

The primary stimulus for secretion of insulin is glucose (sugar).
Insulin and glucagon are the major hormones involved in the control of energy metabolism and they have opposing functions.

Insulin is released to mobilise glucose for use and storage,
thereby decreasing circulating glucose levels (lower blood sugar).

Glucagon is released in response to low blood sugar and:

• promotes glucose formation from fat stores when more sugar is
required than is currently available
• converts stored glucose (primarily from the liver) into
circulating glucose when necessary

• stimulates lipolysis (breakdown to a form suitable for use) in adipose (fat) tissue.

When balanced, these hormones function together to restore low blood sugar to a normal level. Blood-sugar levels may plummet after sugar consumption as a result of the insulin response. Unlike less-refined carbohydrates with nourishment and fibre intact, sugar and highly refined carbohydrates are released quickly in the digestive tract. Glucose is released rapidly into the bloodstream and is then absorbed by cells to satisfy their energy needs. To handle this overload, your pancreas releases large quantities of insulin. This hormone is your body's mechanism for sending glucose into the cells. The problem lies in the quantity of insulin released. If too much sugar is detected at one time, large quantities of insulin are released – often more than are required. As a result, your blood-sugar level drops from too high to too low, creating a roller-coaster of energy. This crash in your blood-sugar levels leaves you feeling anxious, jittery and vague, due to glucose deprivation in your brain. Your adrenal glands may react to this situation by releasing 'stress' hormones that cause your liver to pump stored sugar into your bloodstream. Unfortunately, these hormones will also increase anxiety.

With continued overconsumption of refined sugars, your pancreas will eventually become tired and unable to keep up with the demand. When it is no longer able to clear sugar from the blood, hyperglycaemia (high blood sugar), the onset of diabetes, will result.

> Just to clarify: 'hyper' refers to high blood sugar and 'hypo' to low blood sugar.

Avoid refined carbohydrates and allow your body to use stored fat for its intended purpose – as reserve energy.

There is no magic or mystery involved. You need only ask yourself a few questions.

• Why does your body store excess fat? For what purpose does it intend to use it?

• When you consider it logically, why on earth would you consume 70 to 80 per cent of your calories in the form of energy, preventing your body from utilising reserve fuel (body fat) as energy?

• Why do you continue to deprive yourself of essential nourishment and calories if it doesn't have the desired effect of creating a lean, healthy, energetic body? If it's not working, it's time to change.

THE FAT FILES

Living in an overfat society surrounded by all the hype about how evil fat is makes it hard to believe that we don't eat enough fat, but it's true! You know I'm not talking lard and bacon here but 'friendly' fats. We've thrown our diets out of whack by eating highly processed food. Whether your goal is to eat low-fat food, or you're just addicted to junk food, there's a good chance that you're not getting enough of the 'right' fat in your diet. Omega-3 and -6 fats are essential: we must eat them because our body can't produce them itself. Omega 6 is pretty easy to obtain from our food. It is present in most vegetable oils and animal products such as salad dressing, mayonnaise, margarine and associated commercial products. In fact, most people get way too much omega 6 and not enough omega 3. Omega 3 is found in less-common foods such as cold-water fish and certain oils and nuts. It is unstable and easily destroyed by processing and poor storage. Many studies now indicate that omega-3 fats can alleviate and even prevent many common ailments. It has been known to relieve joint pain and inflammation and even promote fat loss. To keep the correct balance, we need to consume about 1 gram of omega 3 for every 1 to 5 grams of omega 6 every day. Unfortunately, recent US studies have indicated that many people are actually having 20 to 40 times more omega 6 than omega 3.

OMEGA 3 AND OMEGA 6 IN FOODS

FOOD	QUANTITY	OMEGA 3	OMEGA 6	CALORIES
flaxseed oil	1 tablespoon	7.5 g	1.8 g	120
flaxseeds	1 tablespoon	2.2 g	0.5 g	59
fresh salmon	100 g	1.5 g	0.6 g	231
fresh tuna	100 g	1.5 g	0.3 g	128
walnut oil	1 tablespoon	1.4 g	7.5 g	120
cod liver oil	1 tablespoon	2.7 g	0.9 g	123

All the above values are based on unrefined products. The omega value can change significantly if a food is exposed to heat, light, oxygen or any excessive processing.

ALTERED FATS

Margarine is one of the most perfect examples of altered fat I can think of. It is most commonly manufactured from cottonseed oil, maize (corn) oil or soya bean oil.

Many margarines contain trans-fatty acids and partially hydrogenated oils. Trans-fatty acids can lower levels of HDL (good) cholesterol and raise levels of LDL (bad) cholesterol (see 'What Are You *Really* Eating?' in Chapter 5).

The frightening thing about all of this is that there is now a whole generation (or two) that has been raised with margarine as part of its staple diet. I shudder to think of the damage this has done. A new generation of margarines is claiming to contain 'no trans-fatty acids or partially hydrogenated fats'. Some are actually claiming to include omega 3 fats. I'm not sure how these are incorporated into the spread. However, I think manufacturers would have a hard time carefully stirring in unrefined fresh flaxseed oil after the product had been manufactured. This is the only way I know to preserve the goodness in omega 3 oils. When you've finally finished reading the margarine's long list of ingredients and additives, you'll probably make the most sensible decision and put it back on the shelf.

The government of Holland has come to its senses, banning the sale of margarine that contains trans-fatty acids. The Dutch have a higher life expectancy than any other Westerners.

case study sandy

Each time I walked into the gym, there was a woman on the exercise bike pedalling like there was no tomorrow. When I left, an hour later, she was usually still there. A few months later, Sandy came to me for advice. She was desperate to trim down her thighs. She had a petite upper body, yet she could never seem to budge that lower-body fat. Why? After a bit of research, we discovered that Sandy was eating a relatively low-calorie diet and exercising vigorously for 1½ to two hours every day, all to no avail. The problem? She diligently followed a diet almost devoid of fat and very high in refined carbohydrates. Sandy believed that she needed the carbohydrates to provide the energy she needed to complete her exercise. She regularly suffered from symptoms of low blood sugar, including headaches, dizzy spells and nausea. Her energy levels and moods fluctuated dramatically.

After increasing her calorie intake, adding some decent fats and protein to her diet and reducing all of the refined food she ate, Sandy couldn't believe the improvement. Within six weeks there was a visible change in her body composition, creating the more balanced appearance she was striving for. Her episodes of low blood sugar were eliminated within weeks of changing her diet. Sandy's energy and moods seemed to stabilise and she was able to cut her vigorous cycling sessions in half yet still reap the rewards. It just goes to show: more is not always better.

QUESTION   *What can I do to change my body's response, allowing it to burn body fat for fuel?*

ANSWER   • Keep your insulin and blood-sugar levels under control by avoiding refined carbohydrates.
• Consume adequate calories for your BMR.
• Consume the desired 'fat burning' ratio of protein, carbohydrates and fats.
• Be active – you won't burn fuel from any source unless you stimulate the process by moving.

By stabilising your blood-sugar levels and not stimulating the overproduction of insulin, you will enjoy a much happier and healthier existence. When you balance your dietary intake by consuming adequate amounts of protein, essential fats and unrefined carbohydrates, you will become efficient at burning stored fat for fuel. Your body is quite brilliant really. Instead of trying to fight it, learn to respect the way it functions and manipulate the processes you want to work for you.

QUESTION *I do quite a bit of jogging. I need to eat 'high-carb' foods and drink sports drinks to get me through my exercise, or I tend to run out of energy. You would probably recommend against this, wouldn't you?*

ANSWER I don't believe that anyone *needs* to consume high-sugar foods, devoid of nourishment, to provide them with energy! Depending on the intensity and duration of your exercise sessions, I can suggest a couple of things about your diet that might need correction.

• If you are running out of energy, perhaps you are not consuming enough calories in general in your daily regimen. Try increasing your total calorie count by eating more 'real' food.

• Your blood-sugar levels may be fluctuating in the middle of your exercise session due to an imbalance in your ratios of protein, carbohydrates and fats. I would suggest that the very foods you are consuming for energy are responsible for your energy loss. At present, it sounds as though you are attempting to remedy this by continuously fuelling the sugar drip. When you consume sugar-rich food and liquids, your body overproduces insulin, lowering your blood-sugar level too much. When your blood-sugar level drops below the desired level, particularly during exercise sessions, you experience extreme fatigue and perhaps even feel light-headed and dizzy. Once you address your problem by making positive changes to the ratio of the protein, carbohydrate and fat you eat, I'm sure that the necessity for a 'sugar hit' will disappear.

I have always thought that eating fat would make you fat. It sounds logical to me. What do you think?

It's not quite that simple. When you eat fat it doesn't automatically become magnetically attracted to your backside! We often avoid fat simply because we have been brainwashed by 'experts' to think that it's detrimental to our health and weight. Unfortunately, stored fuel in the body and dietary fat have the same name and are, therefore, easily confused. Dietary fat has a higher energy/calorie value than either protein or carbohydrate:

> 1 gram of dietary fat = 9 calories
> 1 gram of carbohydrate = 4 calories
> 1 gram of protein = 4 calories

The logic applied to the 'eat fat and get fat' theory is all related to calories. If you eat low-fat food, the idea is that you will eat fewer calories. Unfortunately, low-fat diets just stimulate us to eat more of the lower-calorie foods. By the end of the day we will usually have broken even or consumed even more energy. If you refer back to the Body Composition chapter (Chapter 2) you can remind yourself why calorie restriction is not the *ideal* way to go. Stored fat is a result of an imbalance in your energy-balance equation. Quite simply, this means you are eating more energy (calories) than you burn (as a result of activity and your BMR).

> If you eat more than you need, whether in the form of carbohydrates, protein or fat, your body will convert it into triglycerides (blood fats) and transport it to the reserve fuel tanks (fat cells) for later use.

As the majority of the population consumes at least 70 per cent of its food in the form of carbohydrates, it makes sense that this, not dietary fat, is the likely 'fat' culprit. Because dietary fat makes us feel full, we tend to eat *more* total calories to compensate when we eliminate or reduce it. Of course, the dietary fats that I am promoting are the healthy ones. I am certainly not justifying the consumption of any highly processed, undesirable fats. Unfortunately, our beloved traditional food pyramid has given us all a 'fat-phobia'. Many of us don't differentiate between the various types of dietary fats, some being essential and healthy, others being quite detrimental to our health. In the ancient, outdated pyramid, all fats and oils are squeezed together in the 'pointy bit' at the top, indicating that we should consume as little as possible! I've never seen the logic in comparing fats from such sources as avocado or nuts with margarine and overused deep-frying oil! If you follow the principles of 'real food' this is almost impossible anyway, as bad fats are associated with the highly processed, sugar-laden foods that you will be avoiding! Surely by now we have enough knowledge to elevate the good fats – or should I say bring the good fats down to a fatter bit of the pyramid!

8

chaptereight

ANTI-AGEING NUTRITION

Are you older than you need to be?

A nyone who lives in the Western world will be aware of the plethora of research and experimentation concerning age-ing and how to slow it down: the search for the eternal fountain of youth.

Much of the latest research indicates that we have a biological age as well as a chronological age. What on earth does this mean? It is simply a way of measuring how well, or how badly, we age.

Your chronological age is, of course, your age in years – how many birthdays you've accumulated, without cheating! Your bio-logical age refers directly to your state of health, in comparison with your years – how much wear and tear your body has been sub-jected to, and how kind the years have been to you. For instance, you may have a chronological age of thirty-two but a biological age of forty-seven. You may laugh, but unfortunately this is an all-too-common reality. A combination of tests is used to compile these statistics, and ultimately they are only estimates. They do, how-ever, give us some indication of how well, or how badly, we have been looking after ourselves so far! Obviously, a certain amount of credit (or blame) belongs to our genetic make-up. Some of you may be blessed with flawless, olive skin (I must have been holding open the door when this was being issued!), others with thick, fabulous hair, and so on.

The rate at which our bodies age, or deteriorate, is well documented. If your biological age surpasses your chronological age, you're not doing very well at all. On the other hand, it is possible for your biological age to be much lower than your chronological age, meaning that you're actually very youthful for your years and are decaying at a much slower rate than some of us.

Jokes aside, you can control, to a degree, the rate at which your body ages. That is the essence of my philosophy – preservation and prevention. Who actually wants to live the last twenty years of their life trapped in a sick, arthritis-ridden, debilitated body? Many diseases today are accepted as part of the normal process of ageing. This is rubbish. They are dubbed 'normal' because they plague a large percentage of the world's population. Perhaps because they are not unusual or uncommon it is considered safe to call them normal.

You have two choices:

• sit back and accept all of the debilitating illnesses of 'natural ageing'

• do all you can to prevent disease and preserve your body by feeding it with the appropriate nourishment, and by avoiding many of the things we know are going to have a detrimental effect; oh, and by the way: you'll look great too.

Many of us will resign ourselves to the fact that the way we age is determined by our genes. Older members of your family may have developed diabetes, heart disease or colon cancer near the end of their life, but I don't believe that this necessarily means that you will too. Sure, we may have genetic tendencies toward certain ailments, but we are all aware of the dramatic effects that diet changes have on diseases. Many male clients have said to me, 'Most of the men in my family have "love-handles", so that's why I have them. It's genetic. I'll never get rid of them.' What a cop-out! Of course you can get rid of them. Don't blame your father, or your great-grandfather on your mother's side. It may be genetic that you happen to have most of your fat storage cells in this area. However, it's up to you whether you fill them up with fat or not. Your poor old dad isn't forcing the wrong food down your throat.

I believe that the same rules apply to genetic tendencies towards disease. If you fail to look after your body and let your health deteriorate it stands to reason that if colon cancer is the weak link in your genetic chain then colon cancer you will probably get!

WHAT ARE ANTI-OXIDANTS?

Despite their relatively high profile in the media over the past few years, there is still widespread misunderstanding about the role of anti-oxidants. Many people have now heard of anti-oxidants, yet most probably couldn't explain what they are or what they do. Well, I hope this explanation makes some sense.

Anti-oxidants are involved in reducing the risk of more than sixty diseases.

> We've all witnessed a piece of fruit turning brown. What happens when you squeeze a bit of fresh lemon juice over it? Lemon juice has been used for generations to stop cut fruit and prepared platters of food discolouring. Lemons contain a high level of anti-oxidants.

Our bodies are susceptible to contact with oxygen in exactly the same way as fruit. There are anti-oxidant nutrients whose function is, just as their name suggests, to help protect our body from oxidative damage, or stop us from going rusty! Anti-oxidants help to stabilise harmful molecules known as free radicals before they harm our cells. Anti-oxidants are quite heroic little devils, actually sacrificing themselves to protect our bodies. They have now been shown to play a role in the prevention of heart disease, certain cancers and other degenerative disorders. If you are a smoker or are exposed to environmental pollutants etc. you will need greater amounts of many of the anti-oxidant vitamins.

The list of nutrients with anti-oxidant properties is ever-increasing; some of the most common ones are listed here. You'll notice that they all come from 'real food'.

Vitamin E Food sources: fresh and unrefined wheat-germ oil, sunflower seeds, almonds, hazelnuts, tuna, avocado etc.

Vitamin C Food sources: citrus fruits, berries, capsicum, kiwifruit, broccoli, cauliflower, cantaloupe, tomato etc. This vitamin protects other anti-oxidants from oxidation. For every cigarette smoked, as much as 25 mg of vitamin C can be depleted from your body. Environmental pollutants and various medications can also have detrimental effects on this vitamin.

Vitamin A Food sources: liver, cod liver oil, cheese, eggs, milk. Vitamin A is particularly effective at scavenging free radicals generated by cigarette smoke, air pollution and fumes.

Betacarotene Food sources: carrots, mango, pumpkin, spinach, cantaloupe, avocado, tomato, broccoli, apricots, peaches, oranges, paw paw, watermelon, green beans etc. Betacarotene is only one of many carotenes. It has many important roles, including protecting our skin against UV damage and protecting the lining of mucous membranes, the stomach and lungs. In the body it is converted into vitamin A as needed. It is found in the pigment of deep yellow, orange, red and dark-green fruit and vegetables.

Another unique anti-oxidant is pycnogenol (pronounced **pik**-nuh-je-nol). It is an extract of French maritime pine trees. It is rich in bioflavonoids, usually found in abundance in fresh fruits, vegetables, nuts, seeds and whole grains. (However, the fact that it is a very effective and potent anti-oxidant doesn't mean that it is the only one you need to consume for optimum protection. Anti-oxidants work as a team, replenishing one another as they go.)

On a more superficial note, and one that may interest us even more than what's happening on the inside, pycnogenol can protect our skin from rapid ageing and sun damage, help to prevent varicose veins and spider veins, remedy easy bruising and help to heal psoriasis. It's pretty good stuff, huh?

One of the more surprising anti-oxidants is cholesterol. It actually helps to protect our cells against free-radical damage. I'm convinced that health benefits seen following a reduction of cholesterol foods in the diet are likely to be due to the decrease in processed fats and the associated reduction in the risk of oxidisation and free-radical damage. Anti-oxidant properties have also been found in numerous minerals, selenium, zinc, co-enzyme Q10 etc.

WHERE CAN I GET ANTI-OXIDANTS?

You can obtain anti-oxidants from certain foods listed in this chapter, through supplementation or through both. Many anti-oxidants are found in abundance in fresh fruit and vegetables. A diet rich in these foods will provide you with a certain amount of your dietary requirement, depending, of course, on what your individual requirement is. Vitamin E is a little more difficult to obtain from food, particularly for those following a low-fat diet. Vitamin E is a powerful anti-oxidant found in vegetable oils, nuts, seeds, avocado and other fat-rich foods. It is virtually impossible to get enough naturally without overdosing on calories.

Now don't even think for one minute that you can go to the health-food shop and load up with anti-oxidants then go and smoke yourself stupid. You will have a hard enough time trying to replenish your supply after normal bodily demands without significantly increasing the demand deliberately.

WHAT ARE FREE RADICALS? THEY SOUND LIKE SOME SORT OF POLITICAL MOVEMENT!

> Free radicals are destructive little critters that are floating around your body as you read this book!

Okay, critters isn't the scientific term for them; rather, these are molecules of oxygen. To put it simply, a stable molecule would have pairs of electrons but free radicals are missing an electron and their mission is to find one. The only way to get it is to *steal* it from a healthy 'paired' cell. Hence free radicals are basically little biological terrorists, scavenging and wreaking havoc within your body, destroying your healthy cells and damaging valuable tissue in the process. The degree of damage inflicted is dependent on the amount of available anti-oxidant protection you have (i.e. how much *good stuff* you've eaten).

As a result of free-radical attack, the ageing process may be accelerated. Skin loses elasticity, hair thins, muscles weaken, teeth decay, immunity decreases and degenerative diseases surface.

Free-radical production can be caused by oxygen, environmental pollutants, ozone from electrical appliances, UV radiation from the sun, food additives, cigarette smoke, radiation, stress or trauma (either emotional or physical), poor diet, excess alcohol consumption, illness and infection and exposure to heavy metals (including your dental fillings).

Before you decide to eliminate yourself from the category of those at risk, read on. After all, how on earth could you ever be exposed to heavy metals? Here you go:

Lead certain plastics, water, insecticides, porcelain enamel, paint pigments (may be inhaled), candle wicks

Mercury amalgam in dental fillings, large fresh fish (because they consume the smaller fish, increasing concentration of heavy metals), grains treated with mercury fungicide, fabric softeners, floor wax; occurs naturally in the environment but is also spewed into the air by power plants burning fossil fuel then finds its way to our soil and can eventually end up in the ocean

Aluminium antacids, deodorant, buffered aspirins, many processed foods, cookware.

Your body will produce free radicals constantly as it goes about its daily business. The problem arises when you produce too many free radicals and lack the anti-oxidants to neutralise them. This will happen if you expose yourself to the free-radical stimulants mentioned above and don't feed yourself sufficient anti-oxidants. See – your mother was right when she told you to eat your veggies but not when she told you to eat your crusts. Free radicals can also alter protein and DNA, making you susceptible to ailments such as irritable bowel syndrome, auto-immune disease and even cancer.

SUGAR CAN MAKE YOU OLD BEFORE YOUR TIME

Excessive consumption of simple/refined carbohydrates can accelerate the ageing process. How? Through a process known as glycosylation, or cross-linking.

When you consume too many refined carbohydrates and sugars, they can attach themselves to proteins and make them stiff, or rigid. These proteins can be found in your skin, connective tissue or arteries, causing loss of elasticity, impaired function or early signs of ageing.

case study barbara

Barbara loathed the thought of her body deteriorating with age. At fifty-four years old, she is living proof that caring correctly for your body and feeding it the necessary nutrition can retard the process significantly. Even before Barbara read *Fat or Fiction*, she was a devotee of anti-oxidant vitamins accompanied by 'real food'. Having always been an active person, Barbara had an excellent body composition. She managed to maintain a body-fat reading of 24 per cent while never feeling the need for 'fad' diets or radical eating programs. Barbara has followed very similar principles to mine for almost fifteen years. She is adamant that her youthful complexion and good health are primarily due to her lifestyle.

When it comes to the subject of anti-ageing, you'll find that most people above the age of thirty will prick up their ears and stand to attention. Why? Probably because they have discovered that they are not invincible. We have all experienced some signs of ageing by this time and usually we don't like what we see. (Or more importantly, what they can't see.) Personally, I have found that the carefully planned use of anti-oxidant vitamin supplements and avoidance of free-radical triggers (when possible) works a treat. I intend to fight the ageing process all the way, but there is no magic potion, despite what the cosmetic companies tell us: if there were, I'd be bathing in it.

QUESTION   *I'm thirty years old and have always eaten exactly what I want – especially junk food. I'm perfectly healthy, I don't exercise and I don't have a problem with my weight, so why should I change anything?*

ANSWER   Congratulations! The only question *I* have for *you* is, 'What defines "healthy"?' Is it being slim? Is it the absence of disease symptoms? Or is it considering yourself to be *fitter* than your peers? We all have our own scale by which we measure ourselves. The question becomes, 'Compared to what or whom?' You have obviously not experienced any major debilitating illness and your current state of health must be sufficient to accommodate your lifestyle, so far. But even a clean bill of health from a medical practitioner only indicates that you have no visible symptoms of the diseases he tested you for. I consider this a far cry from optimum health.

If you are not very active, then you don't really require a very high level of fitness to perform everyday tasks. If you were to raise the demand you put on your body, whether deliberately or through unforeseen circumstances, you might not have a lot in reserve. It's like having a car that sits in the garage. It can be in very poor mechanical condition, but if you rarely drive it, you'll probably never notice. If you had to take it out for a decent drive one day, you'd probably realise that it was in desperate need of some TLC. The major problem you may encounter at some stage of your life will be the result of the unseen deterioration your body may be accumulating, or the long-term effect that can result from inadequate nourishment. Even if you think you are invincible at the moment, your body will only take so much abuse before it is overwhelmed and breaks down. Because it is the only body you will ever have, and it has to last you a lifetime, I would highly recommend treating it with the utmost respect. That way, it might last the distance.

QUESTION *Can I get all the anti-oxidants I need from my food or do I need to take supplements?*

ANSWER This is such a hard question to answer broadly. Everybody's requirements are so very different. Many factors come into play when it comes to nutritional requirements, particularly when we're talking about anti-oxidants. These requirements are also very changeable, depending on our current lifestyle demands. Some influencing factors may be:

stress levels physical exercise or emotional trauma
recovery from illness, disease or surgery
environment inhaling pollutants, passive smoking etc.
smoking
food the quantity of chemicals and additives in our food chain
calorie restriction inadequate nourishment from food, through weight loss attempts or poor food choices.

Even if we attempt to eat all the right foods, quite often the food itself is not of high quality. Many natural foods are produced in undesirable environmental conditions, including depleted soils. They might then be incorrectly packaged, stored and transported. It's really not made very easy these days to obtain all the required nutrients from our food. For this reason, I *do* think that it is necessary to take supplemental anti-oxidants. Find a broad-spectrum anti-oxidant tablet and make sure it is of the highest potency and contains the largest range of anti-oxidants available.

You will probably find that your health-food shop will be able to assist you in choosing the most appropriate one, if you specify these requirements. GNC is an American health-food shop franchise now operating in Australia. I do recommend them to my clients because all the staff are qualified naturopaths, with a comprehensive knowledge of their merchandise. If there is not a store nearby, you will find them on the Internet. I make mention of this because I know from experience how frustrating and confusing supplement shopping can be. The sheer volume of little bottles on the shelves is daunting. It's just nice to know that there is someone who knows their *stuff*.

HAVE WE ALL
GONE MAD?

the power of television

On a recent trip to the USA, I was mesmerised by the never-ending flow of diet-related commercials. The main message being portrayed seemed to be, 'Do nothing and achieve the results you've always wanted, really fast! All you need to do is pick up the phone and dial 1-800. If you can't afford it, we have an easy three-step payment plan, just for you!'

The latest of these commercials seems to be about a product that claims to absorb the fat we consume, rendering it calorie-free. Wow, sounds too good to be true, doesn't it? You're right!

The whole scenario is quite comical really. They front the commercial with a man in a white coat talking a lot of medical mumbo jumbo to establish credibility. This is followed by lots of brightly coloured illustrations of cute little sponges that go around mopping up all the big 'fat' globules, depicted as nasty monsters.

I'd actually like the opportunity to produce a more 'true to life' cartoon of my own, though I'm not sure the manufacturers of these products would like it to go to air. Picture this: The little cartoon character eats a couple of iced jam doughnuts, flooding his stomach with loads of fat globules and sugar. He knows it's bad for his health to eat these foods, but what the heck, he'll now purge them with a magic pill. It's almost like being bulimic, but *it's recommended by doctors*. The magic pill will now bind with the fat he has consumed, taking it through his intestinal tract at great speed, complete with any fat-soluble vitamins, creating a very undesirable *leaky bowel* at the end of its journey. Oh, whoops, didn't they mention that in the ad? Oh well, is leaching your body of essential nourishment and persevering with a leaking rear-end such a price to pay for being able to scoff down high-calorie, nutritionally empty food?

Getting back to the real world, do you understand how crazy this is? Can you imagine what someone from an underprivileged country might think of our strange, gluttonous behaviour? Think about it.

9

chapternine

FIBRE

Why is fibre important for fat loss and good health?

The evolution of food processing and the modern-day diet has led to a more refined food chain, and with it, a severe lack of natural fibre. A correlation has been shown to exist between a low-fibre diet and many diseases. An increase in fibre intake can prevent, or even reverse, detrimental effects of some medical conditions. From ailments such as constipation, haemorrhoids, gallstones and high cholesterol to ulcers and varicose veins, a lack of essential fibre may be the villain.

GRAINS

Grains such as wheat, corn and rice are the most commonly consumed crops in the world. Knowledge of their consumption goes back over 10 000 years. Whole, unprocessed grains provide a healthy amount of B vitamins, vitamin E and numerous minerals, essential to good health. With all this goodness, you may think I'm mad for not highly recommending the consumption of cereals, bread and pasta. Let me explain a few facts about food processing, and what actually happens to our precious grains.

The Endosperm: the central core (approximately 80 per cent of the grain)

The endosperm is the part of the wheat that flour is made from. It is composed of starch (minimal protein) and is used as energy to nourish the future seed. It contains nourishment to help the seed grow. However, it has fewer B vitamins and minerals than the germ and bran, which are removed in processing.

The Germ: the future sprout (approximately 3 per cent of the grain)

Although small, the germ is an essential part of the grain. It can be likened to the foetus: it is nourished by the placenta (endosperm) and protected by the womb (bran). It contains protein, oils and many vitamins and minerals. When processed, the germ is broken apart, allowing the deterioration of the nourishment and oils contained within.

The Bran: the outer covering (approximately 15 per cent of the grain)

This serves as a protective coating and contains much of the fibre and nutrients. One advantage of removing the outer bran coating when processing grains is that it contains a high percentage of phytic acid. This can bind essential minerals when ingested, rendering them useless. Many people who resort to bran supplements to compensate for poor dietary habits may increase their risk of mineral depletion. Adding high-fibre whole foods to your diet is a far more desirable way to ensure adequate fibre intake.

THE DANGERS OF EATING TOO MANY GRAINS

There are sound reasons for ensuring you don't eat too many grains.

- Refined grains lose the mineral zinc in the outer casing, creating a mineral imbalance.
- If not kept refrigerated, whole grains and their by-products, such as wheat germ, may go rancid. Once the outer bran is disrupted or the grain is refined, it slowly decays.
- Many people consume grains that are less than perfect, resulting in incomplete digestion and the development of allergies.

WHAT ABOUT RICE?

Unfortunately, most commercially available rice is refined, or polished. Removing the outer bran layer would still leave most of the nourishment in tact. Unfortunately, further processing usually takes place. The rice is bleached, cleaned, polished with talc and oil coated. Due to this processing, oils are lost, protein reduced and up to 80 per cent of the B vitamins destroyed, along with many minerals.

ESTION   *Aren't high-fibre foods also high-carbohydrate foods?*

ANSWER   They can be. However, some of the best sources of fibre are quite low in carbohydrates. Many undesirable high-carbohydrate foods are highly processed and sadly lacking in fibre anyway. The first foods we think of when fibre is mentioned are probably cereals, bread and rice. The table on page 106 gives you a few examples of desirable sources of fibre:

FIBRE AND CARBOHYDRATE CONTENT OF FOODS

SOURCE	FIBRE (g)	CARBOHYDRATE (g)
WHOLE FOODS		
1 passionfruit	3	3
1 tomato	3	5
½ avocado	2	5
1 nectarine	2	6
1 cup bean sprouts	3	2
½ cup broccoli	4	3
1 cup cabbage	2	2
½ cup cauliflower	3.3	2
25–30 almonds	4.3	1
2 tablespoons flaxseeds	6	1
1 tablespoon tahini paste	2	4
30 g sesame seeds	8	1
COMMERCIALLY MARKETED 'FIBRE-RICH' FOODS		
muesli bar (average)	5	55
1 slice multigrain bread	1.4	14
1 cup Nutri-grain cereal	1.5	21.5
1 cup cooked spaghetti	3	37
1 cup cooked white rice	1.2	42
1 cup cooked brown rice	2.4	48

Don't forget that I am only addressing the fibre content of the abovementioned foods. Although whole foods win this debate hands down, when the values of other nutritional elements are compared, it only confirms that there is no contest.

Are there different types of fibre I need to consume?

Yes, there are two main types of fibre, 'soluble' and 'insoluble', each with quite different functions – just another reason to consume a variety of real, whole foods. This really is the easy way out of attempting to calculate every morsel of food you eat. It doesn't have to get complicated – just choose *real, unprocessed* foods and everything else will fall into place. I cannot say this often enough: consumption of fibre-depleted foods and drinks can hinder weight-loss efforts, as they are a far more concentrated form of calories and easy to overconsume.

For optimum health, you should consume between 30 and 40 grams of combined fibre sources every day. Fibre has many functions, including:

- providing bulk to fill the stomach, satisfying appetite
- helping to regulate the transit time of food in the digestive tract, preventing constipation
- regulating the release of sugars from our food
- assisting regulation of blood cholesterol levels
- assisting weight control
- perhaps helping to prevent colon cancer.

Soluble fibre is found in fruit, vegetables, oat bran, psyllium husks and flaxseeds. It is usually found inside the plant cells. This fibre forms a 'gel' when ingested, helping to control blood-sugar levels and sustain a feeling of satiety.

The best sources of insoluble fibre are wheat bran, whole grains, nuts, seeds and the skin of fruit and vegetables. It usually makes up the structural part of plant cell walls.

HAVE WE ALL
GONE MAD?

the wonders of modern medicine

A couple of years ago, my husband was admitted to hospital in the USA with acute appendicitis. We were in the Bahamas when he was diagnosed with a white-blood-cell (WBC) count of 18000 (normal is around 4000), indicating that his immune system was attempting to fight an acute infection. We immediately flew to the closest 'civilised' medical centre in Fort Lauderdale, Florida. Nobody seemed able to diagnose the cause of his high WBC count and abdominal pain, but appendicitis seemed the most likely cause. After hours of CAT scans and blood tests, a surgeon and a gastroenterologist decided that key-hole surgery was the best course of action. At that point, my husband had already spent three days 'nil by mouth' in hospital, anticipating surgery. After the operation, he remained in hospital for a week, due to complications (another story entirely). However, my point is that he had lost 8 kg of body weight over this week. Surely, a very ill person fighting an acute infection doesn't need the added stress of malnutrition? Apart from an intravenous drip supplying him with four different antibiotics and glucose (sugar), he received no other nourishment.

When he was able to ingest 'real food', the hospital staff brought him red jelly and ice-cream.
Great! Some sugar, gelatine, red food colouring,
preservatives and some more sugar - how very nutritious. How does an immune system function with this
type of fuel? The physical stress of surgery, acute
infection and the medication all taxed his energy
reserves, yet he was supplied with practically no
nourishment whatsoever. The rationale of the hospital staff was that he needed 'easy-to-digest foods'.
I asked the surgeon to give him an injection of B
vitamins because of the large volume of antibiotics
being administered intravenously. His comment was,
'No, I don't believe in vitamins.'

10
chapterten

TROUBLESHOOTING
No more excuses

It really is possible to make your diet fit your lifestyle. It's quite easy to pick your way around any meal, selecting the parts you wish to eat and avoiding those you don't.

TAKE-AWAY AND FAST FOOD

I know there are more diet gurus out there than you can poke a stick at. While they don't agree with one another on innumerable issues, there is almost universal agreement on one thing: processed junk food can be detrimental to health and cause excess weight gain. I don't think there are many people who haven't heard this before. Let's face it, we all know it's not good for us, but sometimes it just happens: you are out socially with a group of people who decide to pull into the nearest take-away drive-through. Do you give in to peer pressure and allow yourself to have the largest, greasiest serving you can find? After all, what choice do you have? *Plenty,* is the answer! The preferred take-away foods listed on page 112 are the best of a bad bunch and may get you out of an awkward social situation at some time in the future.

Hungry Jack's Order a grilled chicken burger and diet cola... lose the bun!

Red Rooster Order any variation of barbecue chicken (skin-free); discard the stuffing. Don't even think about those wedges!

KFC Tender roast/barbecue chicken (skin-free) is okay, without chips, potato, gravy, sauces, stuffing or fries.

McDonald's Any burger, minus the bun, is the answer, but no nuggets, sundaes, fries or shakes.

Nando's Any chicken (skin-free) is acceptable.

Pizza Try very hard to convince your friends that pizza is just not very cool. If you fail, eat the topping and use the base as a frisbee.

Sandwiches Choose fillings galore and have them put into a container – no bread. If you're faced with prepared sandwiches, choose the ones with the most acceptable filling and don't eat the bread, or at least not all of it.

DINING OUT

It really couldn't be much easier to choose appropriate food from a menu, and it's quite socially acceptable to boot. Some ethnic menus may put a slightly difficult spin on things. However, I think this is probably the case whether you're being conscious of your diet or not. Generally, most cafes and restaurants will have meat, chicken or fish available, with a choice of salad or vegetables. It's real food. If you were following a low-fat diet, it would be far more complicated. Wouldn't you rather order a fillet steak and a Greek salad with dressing on the side than a dry, skinless steamed chicken fillet with two lettuce leaves? My general rule is that if you can't see the ingredients that have been used, don't eat the dish. For example, avoid curries, casseroles, pies, sauces, dressings, marinades, dips and spreads. This will leave you ordering reasonably plain food, but there is nothing to stop you from adding things like balsamic vinegar, soy sauce or a splash of tomato sauce afterwards. Think of how good you will feel without that stodgy food weighing you down.

Cafe-style Meals

The best choices are salads such as chicken, turkey, beef, tuna, salmon and lamb. Ask for the dressing on the side. This way, you can decide whether to add a small amount as you need it or use balsamic vinegar instead. Sometimes a Caesar-style salad will be served with a poached egg on top. If softly poached, it makes a great dressing substitute. Often, sandwich shops have the ingredients set out ready to create a sandwich with requested fillings. It is not unusual to ask for your favourite sandwich fillings to be placed in a plastic container or on a plate for you (e.g. salad greens, hard-boiled egg, cheese, meat, chicken or fish, tomato and cucumber.)

Chinese

This is one of the more difficult menus to choose from because a wide variety of sauces and marinades are used in Asian-style cooking. If faced with such a menu, you will just have to order chicken, meat or seafood, served with plain combination vegetables. Some form of omelette would be another option. Avoid the fried rice, spring rolls, dim sims, prawn crackers, wantons, noodles, sweet and sour sauce, black bean sauce, oyster sauce and plum sauce, not to mention the fried ice-cream balls. But lucky you: you can have the fortune cookie. Break it open, take out the paper, read your fortune and throw the rest away.

Italian

When we think Italian, many of us think pasta. Believe it or not, Italian menus are usually the easiest of them all. I have yet to come across an Italian restaurant that doesn't have an *easy* menu. Obviously, you will avoid the pastas, lasagne, ravioli, spaghetti, cannelloni, gnocchi, minestrone, pizza, garlic and herb bread, and won't even think about the gelati and tiramisu. Try steak, chicken or fish with a large salad or vegetables . . . yum!

Indian

This is a very awkward menu that I would try to avoid whenever possible. Much traditional Indian cooking revolves around heavy sauces and these go against my policy of only eating food if you can see all the ingredients. If eating Indian is unavoidable, I can only suggest that you choose a meal as plain as possible from the selection on the menu. However, if the event is being organised by a group of friends, I'd definitely plead 'allergic tendencies' to try persuading them to go elsewhere.

Japanese

This one is a cinch! Avoid rice, sushi and tempura. Choose from sashimi (raw fish), teppan yaki, some omelettes (depending on ingredients), nori (seaweed), tofu, vegetables and miso soup.

Lebanese and Greek

Choose from beef, lamb, shish kebab, salad and vegetables. Avoid pastries, tabouli, rice, hummus, falafel, couscous, baklava and yiros.

Mexican and Spanish

These are awkward menus to select from. I recommend that you choose salsa, chilli and beef dishes and avoid taco shells, nachos, beans, corn chips, burritos, fajitas and paella.

Vietnamese and Thai

Choose beef, fish or other seafood, chicken or pork served with assorted vegetables, prepared as simply as possible. Have ingredients stir-fried or steamed, or choose a traditional salad – the less fancy, the better. Avoid spring rolls, satays, heavy sauces and coconut dishes, rice, noodles and curry.

TRAVELLING

On an aeroplane your choices are limited.

- You can take your own food, such as raw nuts, pieces of fresh fruit or small containers of fruit in natural juice with no added sugar and protein bars (read the labels and make sure they contain no more than 15 grams of carbohydrates per bar).
- Take a chance and select what you can from the food you're given. Even though this can be done quite successfully sometimes, it is a little risky unless you have some backup food in your hand luggage. Always carry a large bottle of water in your bag. Many travellers don't drink enough water during long flights, increasing jet-lag symptoms tremendously.

Just remember, you are sitting on your backside, sometimes for many hours if you're flying internationally. You probably won't need a great deal of fuel anyway.

Make sure that you consume a lot of fresh water. Avoid the alcohol and limit coffee, tea, diet cola and other caffeine-based beverages. Try to avoid salty foods, as they will increase fluid retention.

IN YOUR HOTEL

If you find yourself in a hotel, you will be totally reliant on others to feed you breakfast, lunch and dinner on a daily basis. Even so, you can stick to this program – I do it myself regularly.

Breakfast

• Omelettes (or egg-white omelettes) filled with cheese, mushroom, tomato, onion, spinach, capsicum etc. and with a grilled tomato on the side.

• Fresh seasonal fruit plate with either cheese, cottage cheese or plain yoghurt. If you have a protein powder sachet with you, mix this into your yoghurt, or make a protein shake.

• Poached or scrambled eggs with grilled tomatoes.

Lunch and Dinner

• Most hotels will accommodate you with room-service menus or will have in-house restaurants. Whether you are dining in the hotel complex or in an independent restaurant/cafe, you can refer back to the 'Dining Out' section in this chapter for menu ideas.

ALCOHOL CONSUMPTION

'Moderation' is the word I like to use when it comes to the subject of alcohol consumption. I realise that there are probably more interpretations of this word than I care to acknowledge. However, I'll attempt to give you some guidelines that, hopefully, won't become too distorted!

The best choices of alcoholic beverages are dry wines – preferably reds. If choosing spirits, be wary of mixers. Soda or diet mixers are preferable. Even tonic water is full of calories and sugar.

Avoid cocktails containing sugar, liqueurs, syrups, cordials, juices and cream – this should cover 99.9 per cent of them. Beer is not a good choice and wine coolers and premixed spirits in cans are shockers. Liqueur coffees are far from desirable, as are punch and fruit drinks. Champagne is designed for celebrations: try and save it for those occasions.

A glass or two of wine with your evening meal a few times per week is fine. Drinking every night is pushing the boundaries of moderation somewhat.

Just to give you some concept of the amount of excess calories one can consume by drinking alcohol, I have listed a few favourites here. For some, a glass of one of these is equivalent to an entire extra meal.

CALORIES AND KILOJOULES IN ALCOHOLIC DRINKS

DRINK	CALS	KJ
pina colada	290	1210
white Russian	370	1545
grasshopper	420	1755
brandy Alexander	370	1545
red wine (average glass)	80	335
amaretto (30 ml)	110	460
Baileys (30 ml)	95	400
Irish coffee (average)	190	795
average spirits (30 ml)	66	275
bottle of beer (4.9% alcohol)	280	1170
bottle of beer (0.9% alcohol)	125	525

SOCIAL OCCASIONS

I guess I have it quite easy in these situations. My friends are so aware of my eating habits that they expect me to be a little different. They either get used to accommodating my strange habits or just avoid inviting me . . . simple.

But seriously, it can be very awkward to be put in a situation in which you are dining at a friend's home and a meal is put in front of you that you simply don't want to eat. I suppose this can happen whether you are watching your diet, or not. I think it's very easy to ask, when you are initially invited to dinner, if your host can just give you the basics without the extras. Chances are, he or she is serving a protein of some kind and some vegetables. At least you're not requesting anything too complicated. I've heard many people say that they didn't want to appear rude or disrespectful so they ate an entire meal to please the host. This comes down to a personal choice – one that I can't decide for you. I can only say that I would not eat something that I didn't want to eat just to gain the approval of somebody else, as I'm sure your friends wouldn't expect you to.

There are very few meals that you couldn't compromise with. Even if you were served a lasagne, you could eat the meat and cheese but leave the pasta sheets; if served pasta bolognaise, you could eat the sauce and leave the pasta. Don't eat the bread on the table and decline dessert, pleading elegant sufficiency. Unless, of course, it's a platter of fresh seasonal fruits and a yummy selection of cheeses.

Anyway, when your friends see the changes in your body shape and energy levels, they'll be bugging you to tell them what *they* should be eating.

HAVE WE ALL
GONE MAD?

family values

Quite recently, I witnessed a seemingly harmless family routine while having lunch at a local cafe. To set the scene: into the cafe walked a family of four – mum, dad and two boys aged eight to ten years old. When their food arrived, the mother, without even glancing up from her magazine, handed her plate across to one son. The boy proceeded to scrape his salad onto his Mum's plate and shovel the chips from her plate onto his own. He was left with a large piece of deep-fried battered fish, a large serving of chips and a contented smile, having cleaned away the green poison.

Not a word was uttered during the exchange. This was obviously a familiar ritual. The younger of the two boys declined lunch without contest, deciding on just a cola to wash down the rest of his bag full of lollies. Yes, there's nothing like a soft drink containing tablespoons of liquid sugar to wash down that bag of solid sugar – what a great lunch for a growing, active child. I'm certain that the two boys will embrace these habits, adhere to them throughout their lives and hand them down to their children.

A scary thought, wouldn't you agree?

11

chaptereleven

WHAT ABOUT ARTIFICIAL SWEETENERS?

The bittersweet reality

There are many raging arguments today concerning artificial sweeteners. It seems as though it doesn't matter what we eat, or what new invention they come up with, it turns out to be bad for us. Since my first book, I've had several comments about the fact that I use sweeteners instead of sugar in many recipes. 'Isn't it bad for us?' many disillusioned readers have asked. The following information should shed some light on the subject of sweeteners and, I hope, put your mind at rest. Although I do recommend using certain sweeteners in some sweet recipes, as well as in tea and coffee, I don't recommend consuming them in large amounts. Sure, there is quite a lot of sweetener in some of the recipes in *Fat or Fiction*. However, I have never intended these 'sweet treats' to be consumed in large quantities on a daily basis. Some readers have said, 'But there is 50 grams of artificial sweetener in each batch of chocolate fudge balls!' Yes, but the recipe will make at least twenty-five balls (2 grams of sweetener in each), of which I recommend you have one or two as a treat. I don't expect you to consume it in place of meals.

WHAT IS IT, AND IS IT SAFE?

Following is information about some of the most common artificial sweeteners.

Sucralose (Splenda)

Splenda is the brand name for the sweetening substance sucralose. It is made from sugar through a process that replaces three of sugar's hydrogen-oxygen groups with chlorine atoms. This makes the resulting molecule about 600 times sweeter than sugar. It will not break down or lose sweetness during cooking as many other sweeteners do. Splenda is unable to be broken down by your body's digestive enzymes and therefore has no calorie value. It doesn't have the bitter aftertaste of some sweeteners because it is derived from sugar. Splenda has passed hundreds of tests over many years to gain its approval. It has been declared safe by many regulating authorities around the world. It is not broken down by the body and doesn't react with other substances to create any negative side effects that I am aware of. Any calories present in packaged forms of Splenda are due to the presence of ingredients necessary to add bulk, so it can be used like sugar. Maltodextrin is one such substance. Granular forms of Splenda have two calories per teaspoon, as opposed to the sixteen calories of an equivalent amount of sugar. Many commercial products now contain Splenda – for example baked goods, jelly, yoghurt, sauces, toppings, salad dressings, chewing gum, beverages and confectionery.

Aspartame (NutraSweet and Equal)

The brand names Equal and NutraSweet are ones we are all aware of. Aspartame consists of three molecules joined together:

phenylalanine (50 per cent), an amino acid/protein component found in food; aspartic acid (40 per cent), also an amino acid found in food; and methanol/methyl alcohol (10 per cent), which is also called wood alcohol.

Most supporters of this sweetening substance will respond to concerns by observing that the three components (mentioned above) are found in many natural foods: the amino acids aspartic acid and phenylalanine are found in protein-rich foods while methanol is found in fruit and vegetables. This is true, but the methanol in natural foods is usually in a bound form and the human body doesn't have the enzyme capacity to break it down. Therefore, naturally occurring methanol is not absorbed into the bloodstream. A potential problem with aspartame is that the methanol in it is in 'free form'. In other words, it seems that it can be absorbed. In recent years, I have used particular artificial sweeteners in various recipes, and as a general substitute for sugar in tea, coffee etc. In view of recent controversy about aspartame, however, my advice is that you do some research about the various artificial sweeteners (there are many web sites devoted to the subject) and draw your own conclusions.

The recent controversy has most probably arisen as a result of an increase in the amount of artificial sweetener used in commercial products. I feel that the danger we are facing is that we may find ourselves consuming more than a reasonable quantity without being aware of it. So read those labels and know what you're eating.

Stevia

Stevia is the latest product on the market. At the time of compiling this information, stevia was approved in the USA for use as a commercial sweetening substance and seemed likely soon to be approved in Australia and numerous other countries. *Stevia rebaudiana* is a herb in the chrysanthemum family that grows wild as a small shrub in parts of Brazil and Paraguay.

During the sixteenth century, conquistadors in South America learned of stevia from the local Indians. There are indications that stevia has been used as an additive in teas and medicine since pre-Columbian times. However, a botanist named Antonio Bertoni first recorded its use by native tribes in 1887. By 1931, it was being crystallised for use in food, beverages and pharmaceuticals.

Precise figures on the quantities used around the world are unknown, but it is estimated that Japanese consumers used the equivalent of 700 metric tonnes of these leaves in 1987 alone.

In Japan, stevia has been used in sugar-free versions of chewing gum, yoghurts and even diet cola. It has been used to sweeten Japanese pickles, dried seafood, fish and meat products, confectionery and a variety of other products. The crude stevia leaves and green herbal powder are reported to be ten to fifteen times sweeter than table sugar. The refined extracts (steviosides) are claimed to be 200 to 300 times sweeter. Stevia can be used successfully in cooking and baking. Because it is a relatively new product in this country, I will reserve my judgement. From the information I have gathered to date, it certainly seems like a reasonable alternative to sugar, with no known adverse side effects.

Sorbitol

This is a common sweetening substance manufactured synthetically and used as a sugar substitute in many commercial products. In its natural form, sorbitol is found in berries, plums, apples, apricots, pears and cherries. Excessive consumption of synthetic sorbitol can cause diarrhoea and intestinal cramping. It is used as a moistening agent in many processed foods (particularly in sugar-free lollies and gum) as well as in many cosmetics, toothpaste and various toiletries.

parttwo

menus and recipes

12

chaptertwelve

YOUR PERSONAL SEVEN-DAY MENU PLANNER

You asked for structure . . . well, here it is!

The following seven-day menu planner has been designed to suit your personal body composition. To use this chart effectively, all that you are required to do is have your body composition tested. Once you have established your lean body weight (LBW), choose your category (group A to F – see the following LBW category chart) and use the menu planner to discover what you should be eating. Obviously, there is a range of 10 kg of body weight in each category: the amounts quoted in the table have been calculated to suit the average of this range. If you are at the lower end of the scale in your group, then common sense will tell you that if you are in doubt you should lean towards the lower end of the calorie choice. For example, whenever cheese is suggested, those at the lower end of their weight range should choose reduced fat, while those at the higher end should choose full fat. All meat quantities are raw weights unless otherwise stated.

There are additional recipes in Chapter 14. The LBW information provided with each of them will enable easy substitution of those recipes for recipes in the seven-day menu planner.

LBW CATEGORY

CATEGORY	LBW (KG)	CATEGORY	LBW (KG)
A	35–44	D	65–74
B	45–54	E	75–84
C	55–64	F	85–94

case study bronwyn

I had a letter from a very excited client, informing me that her cholesterol had dropped from 7.4 to 5.5 after five months of following the diet I had given her. Bronwyn's main goal was always to alleviate several health concerns – high cholesterol being one of them. Much to her surprise, many other ailments such as dry, flaky skin, high blood pressure and eczema disappeared. One concern she had was that for the past four weeks her skin had started to develop pimples. At thirty-nine years old, this was not a case of teenage acne. We discovered that the flaxseed oil she had been taking had been left out of the fridge for a few days and had become rancid. When this was replaced with a fresh bottle, Bronwyn's skin cleared up within a week.

DAY ONE

	Group A	Group B	Group C	Group D	Group E	Group F
Breakfast						
protein porridge (see recipe page 157)						
Snack						
raw almonds	40 g	50 g	60 g	70 g	80 g	90 g
Lunch						
lean chicken meat						
(skinless)	100 g	150 g	175 g	200 g	225 g	250 g
Mediterranean salad (see recipe page 174)						
Snack						
1 apple	small	small	medium	medium	large	large
cheese (full cream)	50 g	60 g	70 g	80 g	90 g	100 g
Dinner						
swordfish or						
tuna steak	100 g	150 g	200 g	230 g	280 g	320 g
vegetable stir-fry (see recipe page 177)						

DAY TWO

	Group A	Group B	Group C	Group D	Group E	Group F
Breakfast						
omelette						
whole eggs	1	1	1	2	2	2
egg whites	2	3	4	4	5	6
cheese	30 g	40 g	50 g	60 g	70 g	80 g
vegetables: unlimited quantities – must have at least two varieties						
(e.g. capsicum, mushroom, tomato)						
Cook omelette in a nonstick pan or electric omelette maker,						
lightly brushed with cold-pressed oil.						
Snack						
yoghurt						
(no added sugar)	200 g	250 g	300 g	350 g	400 g	450 g
strawberries	1 punnet	1 punnet	1 punnet	1 punnet	1 punnet	1 punnet
cantaloupe	–	–	–	1 cup	1 cup	1 cup
Lunch						
tuna-slaw						
tinned tuna (water)	100 g	150 g	200 g	250 g	300 g	350 g
cabbage	200 g	200 g	200 g	250 g	250 g	250 g
carrot, grated	1 cup	1 cup	1 cup	1½ cups	1½ cups	1½ cups
mayonnaise	1 tblsp	1 tblsp	1 tblsp	1 tblsp	1½ tblsp	1½ tblsp
	(30 g)	(30 g)	(30 g)	(30 g)	(45 g)	(45 g)
flaxseed oil	5 ml	10 ml	10 ml	10 ml	10 ml	10 ml
onion, capsicum and/or other grated vegetables if desired						
(Use commercial or homemade mayonnaise – see Ingredient Reference page 140.)						
Snack						
raw mixed nuts	40 g	50 g	60 g	70 g	80 g	90 g
Dinner						
lean eye fillet steak	100 g	130 g	160 g	200 g	250 g	300 g
veggie smash (see recipe page 180)						
snow peas	15 pods	15 pods	15 pods	15 pods	15 pods	15 pods
optional: 1 tblsp low-joule tomato ketchup or 2 tsp mustard						

DAY THREE

	Group A	Group B	Group C	Group D	Group E	Group F
Breakfast						
protein shake						
vanilla protein powder (see Ingredient Reference page 142)						
	35 g	40 g	50 g	60 g	70 g	75 g
frozen raspberries	50 g	75 g	75 g	100 g	100 g	100 g
flaxseed oil	10 ml	15ml	15 ml	20ml	25 ml	30ml
Blend ingredients with water. Add approved sweetener to taste (see pages 121–125).						
Snack						
raw cashews	40 g	50 g	60 g	70 g	80 g	90 g
Lunch						
bolognaise with a twist! (see recipe page 162)						
Snack						
1 apple	100 g	100 g	150 g	150 g	250 g	250 g
full-cream cheese	50 g	60 g	70 g	80 g	90 g	100 g
Dinner						
roast chicken –						
white meat, skinless						
(home cooked or						
rotisserie)	80 g	100 g	140 g	180 g	220 g	250 g
veggie-slaw (see recipe page 179)						

DAY FOUR

	Group A	Group B	Group C	Group D	Group E	Group F
Breakfast						
fruit and yoghurt						
raspberries	50 g	50 g	75 g	100 g	150 g	150 g
strawberries	1 cup	1 cup	1 cup	1 cup	1 cup	1 cup
yoghurt	100 g	150 g	200 g	250 g	250 g	300 g
protein powder						
(mixed into						
yoghurt)	25 g	30 g	35 g	35 g	40 g	45 g
(The yoghurt must have no added sugar. Above quantities are calculated						
using full-cream yoghurt. Add approved sweetener to taste.)						
Snack						
full-cream cheese	30 g	40 g	50 g	60 g	70 g	80 g
raw almonds	25 g	30 g	35 g	40 g	45 g	50g
Lunch						
tuna and cottage dip (see recipe page 169)						
Snack						
fudge (see recipe						
page 185)	2 servings	2 servings	3 servings	3 servings	3 servings	3 servings
raw almonds	20 g	30 g	30 g	40 g	50 g	60 g
Dinner						
warm lamb and avocado salad (see recipe page 166)						

DAY FIVE

	Group A	Group B	Group C	Group D	Group E	Group F
Breakfast						
cottage cheese						
(low-fat, plain)	100 g	120 g	150 g	180 g	200 g	220 g
fresh fruit salad	100 g	120 g	150 g	180 g	200 g	200 g
almonds						
(coarsely chopped)	10 g	10 g	10 g	15 g	20 g	20 g
flaxseed oil	5 ml	5 ml	5 ml	10 ml	10 ml	15ml

Mix all ingredients except nuts in a bowl.

Add approved sweetener to taste and sprinkle chopped nuts over the top.

(Cottage cheese may be replaced with low-fat ricotta if preferred.)

Snack						
hard-boiled egg	1 medium	2 medium	2 medium	2 large	2 large	3 large
tomato	1 medium	1 medium	1 medium	1 large	1 large	1 large
cheddar cheese	40 g	40 g	60 g	70 g	80 g	80 g

Eat individually or chop ingredients into a bowl and sprinkle with

balsamic vinegar and pepper.

Lunch						
roast-beef salad						
lean roast beef						
(cooked weight)	80 g	100 g	130 g	150 g	180 g	200 g
avocado	½ small	½ small	½ small	1 small	1 small	1 small
mixed salad						
vegetables	300 g	300 g	350 g	350 g	400 g	400 g

Dress with balsamic vinegar and lemon juice if desired.

Snack						
1 piece of fruit	1 small	1 small	1 medium	1 medium	1 large	1 large
low-fat yoghurt						
(no added sugar)	200 g	300 g	350 g	400 g	500 g	500 g

Dinner

pork stir-fry (see recipe page 165)

DAY SIX

	Group A	Group B	Group C	Group D	Group E	Group F
Breakfast						
vanilla smoothie						
protein powder						
(vanilla)	30 g	40 g	50 g	60 g	60 g	70 g
low-fat yoghurt						
(vanilla or plain)	100 g	150 g	200 g	200 g	200 g	250 g
flaxseed oil	10 ml	10 ml	10 ml	15 ml	20 ml	20 ml
1 teaspoon of vanilla essence (optional)						

Blend together with approximately 250 ml of water. Add approved sweetener to taste.
(Blend ingredients without water to create a thicker mixture rather than a drink.)

Snack						
raw mixed nuts	40 g	50 g	60 g	70 g	80 g	90 g
Lunch						
salmon-slaw						
drained						
tinned salmon	80 g	120 g	150 g	200 g	240 g	280 g
cabbage,						
shredded	200 g	200 g	200 g	250 g	250 g	250 g
carrot, grated	1 cup	1 cup	1 cup	1 cup	1 cup	1 cup
onion, capsicum and/or other grated vegetables if desired						
mayonnaise	30 g	30 g	30 g	30 g	45 g	45 g

Dilute above quantities of mayonnaise with an equal amount of water.

Snack						
strawberries	1 punnet	1 punnet	1 punnet	1 punnet	1 punnet	1 punnet
cantaloupe	½ cup	½ cup	½ cup	1 cup	1 cup	1 cup
full-cream cheese	40 g	50 g	60 g	70 g	80 g	100 g
Dinner						
burger melts (see recipe page 164)						
additional flaxseed oil						
for salad dressing	5 ml	5 ml	10 ml	10 ml	10 ml	10 ml

Serve with a large green salad tossed in vinegar (any kind) and/or lemon juice.

DAY SEVEN

	Group A	Group B	Group C	Group D	Group E	Group F
Breakfast						
scrambled eggs						
egg whites	3	5	2	3	4	4
egg yolks	1	1	2	2	2	2
grilled tomato	1 medium	1 medium	1 medium	1 large	1 large	1 large
grated light cheese	30 g	40 g	30 g	30 g	50 g	50 g
thinly sliced	or	or	and	and	and	and
smoked salmon	60 g	80 g	50 g	70 g	80 g	90 g

Scramble combined egg (and grated cheese, if indicated) in a nonstick pan, lightly coated with oil or butter. Serve grilled tomato and smoked salmon on the side. Cheese may be melted over grilled tomato rather than used in egg mixture.

Snack						
1 piece of fruit	1 small	1 small	1 medium	1 medium	1 large	1 large
yoghurt – low fat	200 g	300 g	350 g	400 g	500 g	500 g
or full cream	100 g	150 g	175 g	200 g	250 g	250 g

Lunch

chicken and avocado salad

    unlimited salad vegetables (except avocado – see below), with as much variety and

      colour as possible

    lean, skinless

chicken meat						
(raw weight)	100 g	120 g	160 g	200 g	220 g	250 g
avocado	¼ small	¼ small	¼ small	¼ small	¼ small	¼ small
dressing						
flaxseed oil	5 ml	10 ml	10 ml	10 ml	15 ml	20 ml

    vinegar (any kind) and/or fresh lemon juice – unlimited

Snack

mixed raw nuts	40 g	50 g	60 g	70 g	80 g	90 g

Dinner

seafood combination (see recipe page 167)

13

chapterthirteen

INGREDIENT REFERENCE
What your body needs and how to choose wisely

I n this chapter I provide details about some of the ingredients used in my menu planner and recipes.

For information about vitamins and minerals, refer to the chart at the end of the chapter.

ALMOND MEAL

This can be purchased in most supermarkets and health-food and nut retailers. Because it is high in omega 6 fat, it would be better to grind fresh almonds as you need them. As this is not always possible, or desirable, the packaged meal will do.

CHEESE AND YOGHURT

In most cases, I favour full-cream products over skim or fat-reduced varieties. It is a grey area where we must use a bit of common sense. Quite simply, I like full cream because I believe that it fills you up and it tastes better. Of course, gram for gram, it is higher in calories, so if you prefer full cream, just have a little less. The lean weight categories are calculated on an average of each 10-kg range. If you are at the lower end of the scale, I suggest you choose reduced-fat products, or have a little less full cream than specified. Vice versa for the higher end of the range. Always read labels carefully and be aware of products containing added sugar.

FRUIT AND VEGETABLES

Obviously these are seasonal. You will always have a wider variety of tropical fruit in summer than in winter months. I always prefer fresh produce whenever possible. However, you may occasionally substitute *plain* frozen fruit, or canned fruit without additives such as sugar or salt. I often use frozen fruit in protein smoothies to add thickness and texture.

I consider some fruit and vegetables to be better value than others, simply because they contain more nutrition and fibre for the amount of carbohydrate. The higher items with higher starch or sugar content that I suggest you avoid, or at least limit, are potatoes, corn, peas, bananas and grapes. It is probably worth investing in a little carbohydrate-counter booklet, just to be sure.

MAYONNAISE

You have the option of finding a suitable commercial mayonnaise or trying the recipe outlined in the recipe on page 186. If you opt for the commercial one, there are a few things you need to be aware of.

• Choose the brand with the *shortest* list of *natural* ingredients. Mayonnaise should contain egg yolk, oil, mustard and lemon juice as its main ingredients. Avoid added sugar, honey, starch etc.
• Choose a product relatively low in fat. The reason for this is that you can't be sure of the quality of oil used in manufacturing, regardless of its origin (canola, sunflower etc.)
• Be aware that some of the low-fat brands are full of sugar.

NUTS

Always choose raw nuts as opposed to roasted. I know that 'dry-roasted' sounds healthier, but the internal oils of the nuts have been exposed to high temperatures, rendering the fat undesirable.

NUT PASTE

There is quite a wide variety of nut pastes available now. We're all familiar with peanut butter – well, these are similar products. The two major differences are as follows.

• They are derived from other kinds of nuts. They include almond paste; almond, brazil nut and cashew (ABC) paste; and walnut paste.

• They should contain no additives. Most commercial peanut butter contains a long list of ingredients, of which none are very desirable. Nut paste should contain one type of ingredient: nuts!

OATS

The less processing a food has been through the better. You can find many variations of oats on the supermarket shelves. Some will contain sugars, along with other additives. Plain rolled oats are my first choice. Second would be 'quick' or '1 minute' oats. There doesn't appear to be much difference in the nutritional value or carbohydrate or fibre content of the two. Rolled oats have been crushed by rollers and partially precooked to facilitate digestion.

OILS

It is most important to choose the appropriate oils for cooking and for use in uncooked meals. The oils most tolerant to heat are:

- cold-pressed virgin (unrefined) olive oil
- 'high oleic' sunflower or safflower oils (bought from health-food shops)
- butter.

For uncooked meals and salads use any unrefined oil. My preference is always flaxseed oil, due to its omega 3 content.

I have yet to find a suitable oil in the supermarket. The health-food shop will carry a much wider range. Most of these temperature-sensitive oils are kept in the refrigerator so they won't go rancid. Ensure you purchase them from a refrigerated environment.

PROTEIN POWDER

There are so many of these to choose from in your health-food shop. My favourite, based on nutritional value, is whey protein concentrate (WPC). In *Fat or Fiction*, I made reference to this and later discovered that a few readers had confused it with plain whey powder. These are two very different products.

WPC is subjected to a complex process to ensure that the protein is not denatured. The lactose and fats are removed at very low temperatures, with care being taken not to diminish the protein's quality and nutritional value. Maintaining WPC in its natural state is essential to ensure it retains its ability to help strengthen our immune system and fight infection. WPC is currently being used to boost the immune system of AIDS patients.

Whey protein isolate (WPI) is a similar product. It has all the abovementioned properties of WPC but has been further filtered to reduce the lactose and fat content. The protein has also been predigested to enhance absorption.

TAHINI

Tahini is made from sesame seeds and these should be the only ingredient in the paste. There are two varieties.

• In hulled tahini the outer husk of the seed has been removed. Hulled tahini is a light creamy colour.
• In un-hulled tahini the outer husk has been incorporated in the product. It has a much darker, chocolate-brown colour and quite a bitter, strong flavour.

I prefer using hulled tahini.

TINNED FISH

I prefer tinned fish packed in water as opposed to oil or brine. This is not because I disapprove of the calories in the oil-packed varieties but because I can't be sure of the type of oil used in these products and the processing it has endured. If I'm going to have oil, I'd rather have oil of the highest quality. If you prefer the oil-packed varieties, just try water-packed and add your own good-quality oil. There are many tinned tuna products on the shelves with added flavour such as chilli or spices. You will just have to read the label carefully and make a decision according to the list of ingredients added. Brine is simply salt water. I recommend avoiding added salt in food whenever possible. We consume enough in our natural food without adding it unnecessarily. My overall choice is water-packed and, if applicable, salt-reduced.

ALL YOU NEED TO KNOW ABOUT NUTRITION

NUTRIENT	WHY DO I NEED IT?
Vitamin A Betacarotene	• aids in growth and repair of body tissues and the maintenance of healthy, disease-free skin • offers protection to the internal mucous lining of the nose, lungs, throat, mouth, intestines etc. • assists in adequate secretion of gastric juices for digestion • helps build strong bones and teeth • aids in the maintenance of immunity and good eyesight
Vitamin B1 (thiamine)	• assists in starch, sugar and alcohol metabolism • stimulates appetite • keeps nerve cells healthy • helps to maintain muscle tone in the stomach, intestines and heart
Vitamin B2 (riboflavin)	• necessary for the metabolism of protein, carbohydrates and fats • aids in the process of growth and maintenance of healthy skin • acts as an anti-oxidant and requires regular replenishment
Vitamin B3 (niacin/nicotinic acid)	• may help to detoxify the body against narcotics and alcohol • promotes circulation and has been proved to reduce cholesterol • aids in the maintenance of healthy nerves, skin, tongue and tissues of the digestive tract and the synthesis of sex hormones
Vitamin B5 (pantothenic acid)	• stimulates the production of adrenal hormones for healthy nerves and skin • assists the release of energy from food consumed • improves the body's ability to withstand stress • helps to maintain a healthy digestive tract and involved in the synthesis of cholesterol and fatty acids

WHERE DOES IT COME FROM?	SIGNS OF DEFICIENCIES
• vitamin A: liver, cod liver oil, cheese, eggs, butter • betacarotene: the colour pigment of fruit and vegetables, e.g. spinach, carrots, broccoli, tomatoes, peaches, watermelon, cantaloupe, pumpkin	• night blindness, sties and other eye disorders, rough, dry skin, blemishes and premature ageing, weak immune system, bladder infections and brittle nails
• pork, organ meat, brewer's yeast, bran and germ of wheat, nuts, egg yolks, seeds, chicken, meat and fish	• fatigue, appetite loss, low blood pressure, lack of coordination, nightmares, loss of mental alertness, heart irregularities
• liver and other organ meat, pork, cheese, chicken, wheat germ, yoghurt, eggs, brewer's yeast, almonds and fish	• cracks in the corners of the mouth, sore tongue, burning sensation or 'gritty' feeling in the eyes, light sensitivity, oily skin, eczema
• lean meat, poultry, tuna, salmon, swordfish, liver, pork, veal, wheat germ, desiccated liver tables, avocado, sunflower seeds, mushrooms and eggs	• bad breath, fatigue, ulcers, dermatitis, diarrhoea, rough skin, tremors, nervous disorders, insomnia and recurring headaches
• organ meat, brewer's yeast, egg yolks; found in all living cells and widely distributed in yeasts, moulds and bacteria (synthesised in the body by intestinal flora); approximately 33 per cent is lost in the cooking of meat and 50 per cent in the milling of grains	• sensitivity to insulin, upper respiratory infections, skin disorders, low blood sugar and duodenal ulcers (deficiencies may arise due to lack of intestinal flora needed for synthesis)

ALL YOU NEED TO KNOW ABOUT NUTRITION

NUTRIENT	WHY DO I NEED IT?
Vitamin B6 (pyridoxine)	• involved in the release of glycogen from the liver and muscles and therefore essential in physical activity • must be present for the production of blood cells and cells of the immune system • may help to alleviate symptoms of premenstrual tension (PMS)
Vitamin B12 (cobalamin)	• necessary for normal metabolism of protein, carbohydrates and fats, as well as for the regeneration of red blood cells • aids in the maintenance of healthy nerves and mental abilities • aids the body's absorption of carotene, or vitamin A • necessary for the production of haemoglobin and DNA, and assists in the function of iron
Folic acid (folate)	• active in the role of cell division and involved in the formation of red blood cells • necessary for normal brain function and concentrated in the spinal fluid • stimulates hydrochloric acid production, helping to prevent food poisoning and intestinal parasites • aids function of the liver and DNA duplication • may protect against colon cancer
Vitamin C (ascorbic acid)	• strengthens cell and blood-vessel walls • promotes healthy teeth, gums, bones and joints • assists in the formation of collagen and connective tissue • aids wound and burn healing • stimulates the immune system and acts as an anti-oxidant and anti-inflammatory • vitamin C is eliminated in urine and perspiration within three to four hours of ingestion, so regular dietary supply is essential

WHERE DOES IT COME FROM?	SIGNS OF DEFICIENCIES
• organ and muscle meat, tuna, prawns, salmon, egg yolks, nuts, avocado, carrots, wheat bran, sunflower seeds, fresh vegetables, milk and desiccated liver tablets	• anaemia, irritability, weakness, insomnia, skin disorders, hair loss, arthritis, fluid retention and low blood sugar
• organ and muscle meat, eggs, cheese, milk and milk products, fish (animal proteins are the most substantial source of vitamin B12)	• pernicious anaemia, pale skin, fatigue, weight loss, depression, weakness in limbs, diminished reflex response and memory loss
• with a name derived from the word 'foliage', it is not surprising that folic acid is found in green leafy vegetables such as spinach, broccoli, brussels sprouts and cabbage; also found in oranges, liver, brewer's yeast, avocado, wheat bran and almonds (can be destroyed by high cooking temperatures); its antagonists include smoking, alcohol, stress, oral contraceptives and oestrogen	• increased risk of spina bifida in the foetus, anaemia, poor growth, greying hair, metabolic disturbances, forgetfulness and mental sluggishness
• fresh fruit and vegetables such as berries, oranges, broccoli, kiwifruit, capsicum, tomatoes, grapefruit, brussels sprouts, cantaloupe etc.	• shortness of breath, dry skin, impaired digestion, dry and split hair, broken blood vessels, bruising, bleeding gums, nosebleeds, swelling of the joints, anaemia, lowered immune resistance and slow wound-healing

ALL YOU NEED TO KNOW ABOUT NUTRITION

NUTRIENT	WHY DO I NEED IT?
Vitamin D (calciferol)	• involved in the absorption of calcium and promotes its transport in and out of the bones and teeth • necessary for the normal growth of teeth and bones in children • plays a valuable role in the maintenance of a stable nervous system, normal heart action and normal blood clotting
Vitamin E (tocopherol)	• acts as a powerful anti-oxidant • aids in blood-clot prevention • dilates blood vessels, strengthens capillary walls and protects red blood cells • may be beneficial in reducing PMS symptoms, relieving cramping, enhancing immunity, lowering cholesterol and reducing the risk of heart disease and cancer
Vitamin K	• essential in the regulation of blood-clotting to prevent excessive bleeding • plays a role in bone mineralisation and fracture healing • may help prevent osteoporosis
Calcium	• develops and maintains bone structure and rigidity • is involved in the clotting process, nerve-impulse transmission, muscle stimulation, enzyme regulation, vitamin-D metabolism and hormone functions
Chromium	• plays an important role in carbohydrate metabolism • stimulates the enzymes involved in synthesis of fatty acids and cholesterol • increases the effectiveness of insulin, thereby helping to prevent low blood-sugar levels
Iodine	• plays an important role in the development and functioning of the thyroid gland • assists in regulating the body's energy production, promotes growth, stimulates the metabolism and promotes healthy hair, teeth and nails

WHERE DOES IT COME FROM?	SIGNS OF DEFICIENCIES
• those exposed to insufficient sunlight require more dietary vitamin D; other sources include oily fish, such as salmon, mackerel, herring, sardines and tuna, cod-liver oil, egg yolks, butter, cheese and milk-based products	• similar to symptoms relating to calcium deficiency, such as rickets, with symptoms such as bowing legs, poorly developed muscles, nervous irritability, muscle twitching, spinal curvature, softening of the teeth and enlarged wrists, knees and ankle joints
• cold-pressed, unrefined oils, such as wheat-germ oil, safflower oil, soya-bean oil and olive oil, sunflower seeds, almonds, hazelnuts, avocado, spinach, fresh peanut butter, wheat germ, egg yolks and organ meat	• rupture of red blood cells, shrinkage of collagen, muscle wasting and impaired iron absorption
• kelp, alfalfa, cauliflower, leafy green vegetables, cow's milk, yoghurt, egg yolks, safflower oil, fish-liver oils, liver and tomatoes	• defective blood coagulation is one of the only major signs of vitamin-K deficiency; this may manifest itself as haemorrhages, bruising and even miscarriage
• milk, yoghurt, cheese, canned fish with edible bones, shellfish, almonds, broccoli, asparagus, cabbage and sesame seeds	• fragile bones, muscle cramps, rickets, hypertension, abnormal heartbeat, joint pain, increased cholesterol, slow pulse rate, brittle nails, tooth decay and eczema
• brewer's yeast, liver, beef, lamb, meat, cheese and mushrooms	• impaired glucose tolerance and hypoglycaemia (low blood sugar)
• deep-water fish, brown seaweed, kelp, garlic, sesame seeds and spinach (plant and animal sea-life absorb this mineral from seawater)	• goitre (enlarged thyroid gland), hypothyroidism, hardening of the arteries, obesity, lowered metabolic rate, dry hair, rapid pulse, nervousness and irritability

ALL YOU NEED TO KNOW ABOUT NUTRITION

NUTRIENT	WHY DO I NEED IT?
Iron	• essential in the formation of haemoglobin (the red oxygen-carrying pigment in the blood) • increases resistance to stress and disease • improves energy production, growth and oxygen transportation throughout the body
Magnesium	• essential for maintaining a healthy heart, nervous system and muscles • assists calcium in the maintenance of strong bones • is involved in muscle contraction and proper nerve function • may reduce the risk of asthma attacks by relaxing the lining of the lungs • helps to regulate the acid–alkaline balance • promotes the absorption of various nutrients
Potassium	• alongside sodium, aids in the regulation of the fluid balance within the body • essential for muscle contraction, beating of the heart, energy production and protein synthesis • helps to maintain stable blood pressure • stimulates the kidneys to eliminate poisonous body wastes
Selenium	• acts as a powerful anti-oxidant • appears to preserve elasticity of body tissues • works closely with vitamin E in the production of antibodies and binding toxic minerals • assists in maintaining adequate oxygen supply to the heart
Sodium	• helps to regulate the fluid and the acid–alkaline balance within the body • involved in muscle contraction and nerve stimulation • prevents the build-up of other minerals in the bloodstream • involved in oxygen transport and aids digestion

WHERE DOES IT COME FROM?	SIGNS OF DEFICIENCIES
• best sources are liver, oysters and lean meat; second-best sources are leafy green vegetables, whole grains, chicken, strawberries, salmon, tuna, pumpkin, brussels sprouts, almonds, avocado, egg yolks and wheat bran	• anaemia, characterised by symptoms such as constipation, brittle nails, lustreless hair, nail ridges, shortness of breath, lethargy, headache, pale skin, impaired immune response and easy bruising
• green vegetables, seafood, oil-rich seeds, avocado, apples, apricots, wheat bran, salmon, tuna, meat, yoghurt, nuts (especially almonds), garlic, tofu and peaches	• irregular heart rhythm, lack of coordination, muscle twitches, weakness, depression, gastrointestinal disorders, disorientation, confusion, alopecia and swollen gums
• all vegetables, particularly leafy greens, green beans, avocado and pumpkin, sunflower seeds, whole grains, garlic, apricots, apples, cantaloupe, fish, eggs, milk and yoghurt, meat, chicken, tomatoes and raw nuts	• muscular weakness, confusion, irregular heartbeat, poor reflexes, insomnia, constipation, muscle damage, bone fragility and soft, flaccid muscles
• brazil nuts, cashews, fish and shellfish, kidney and liver, fruit and vegetables contain small amounts of selenium, while the content of grains and seeds varies according to the selenium content of the soil in which they were grown	• premature ageing, diminished vision, cataracts, growth retardation, muscular dystrophy and certain forms of cancer; a selenium deficiency may also be implicated in sudden infant death syndrome (SIDS)
• table salt, seafood, kelp, celery, milk, poultry and meat; also present in many processed foods, soy sauce, MSG, nitrate, nitrite, baking soda, spices and other condiments	• gas, weight loss, inability to concentrate, low blood sugar, palpitations and muscle weakness (an excess is more common, with symptoms such as fluid retention, dizziness, high blood pressure and potassium loss)

ALL YOU NEED TO KNOW ABOUT NUTRITION

NUTRIENT	WHY DO I NEED IT?
Sulphur	• assists in maintaining glossy hair and a smooth complexion • sulphur-rich proteins have anti-oxidant properties • assists in formation of collagen (found in bone, skin etc) • is a constituent of the tough protein keratin in our skin, hair and nails • works with the liver to secrete bile (for fat digestion) • may be used topically as an ointment for psoriasis, dermatitis and eczema • the amino acids, including cysteine, contain sulphur and are often given as supplements to improve symptoms of arthritis
Zinc	• plays an important role in immune-system maintenance • improves wound healing • promotes the absorption of the B vitamins • regulates testosterone in the prostate • is a constituent of numerous enzymes involved in digestion and metabolism • is essential in the synthesis of DNA and for the function of taste buds and the skin's oil glands

WHERE DOES IT COME FROM?	SIGNS OF DEFICIENCIES
• concentration in soil determines the quantity found in plant foods – garlic and onions are among the best plant sources; the richest source is eggs, but also present in meat, fish, cheese, milk and soya beans; it's ingested in the form of amino acids (protein)	• deficiencies rare in diets containing adequate protein
• oysters, beef, organ meat, eggs, turkey, lamb, scallops, lobster, pork, whole grains, wheat germ, brewer's yeast, pumpkin seeds, sunflower seeds and nuts	• poor appetite, loss of taste or smell, slow wound healing, susceptibility to infections, excessive hair loss, reduced libido, stretch marks on the skin, white spots on the nails and an irregular menstrual cycle

14

chapterfourteen

RECIPES

Let's create a feast

To make cooking and serving meals on this program as easy as possible, the following recipes are presented in two formats: those that make a single serve that can be multiplied or divided according to your category and those set out in a similar way to the existing recipes in the menu planner. Further information is provided at the start of Chapter 12.

This chapter contains a collection of recipes that my friends, my clients and I have created over the years. You will be amazed at the range of tastes and textures available to you on my program, from delicious omelettes to hearty main meals and mouth-watering treats. They are designed to satisfy your appetite and your cravings, but most importantly, they're actually good for you. Enjoy!

breakfast

FRUIT SALAD SLURPEE

Ingredients

> 1 cup frozen cantaloupe cubes
>
> 1 cup frozen fresh pineapple cubes
>
> pulp of 2 passionfruit
>
> 300 g full-cream natural or fruit-flavoured yoghurt (see pages 48 and 49)
>
> 30 g protein powder (see page 142)

Method

> Remove pineapple and cantaloupe from the freezer and allow to soften slightly. Place all ingredients in a blender and process until fully combined. Spoon into a bowl and serve immediately, or return to the freezer.

> The above recipe is calculated as 1 serving.

Serving size according to your LBW category:

A ½ serving

B ½ serving – top with an extra heaped dessertspoon of yoghurt

C ½ serving – as above, plus extra fruit

D 1 serving

E 1 serving – top with an extra heaped dessertspoon of yoghurt

F 1 serving – as above, plus extra fruit

PROTEIN PORRIDGE

Ingredients

Select ingredient quantities according to your LBW category:

	A	B	C	D	E	F
rolled oats	30 g	40 g	50 g	60 g	70 g	80 g
vanilla protein powder (see page 142)	30 g	40 g	50 g	60 g	70 g	80 g
water						
ground cinnamon						
approved sweetener (optional – see pages 121–125)						

Method

Combine the oats and protein powder in a small nonstick saucepan. Pour over enough cold water to cover dry ingredients (it's better to add less water than necessary, because this allows you gradually to add more during cooking until your porridge reaches a desired consistency). Stir continuously over heat until smooth. When the porridge is cooked to your liking (3–4 minutes), pour into your serving bowl. Sprinkle with cinnamon and/or sweetener

Note: if you prefer to cook your porridge in the microwave, I suggest that you cook the oats in water first, then stir in the protein powder.

THE PERFECT OMELETTE

Ingredients

    2 whole large eggs
    2 egg whites
    30 g parmesan cheese, shredded
    30 g mozzarella cheese, grated
    freshly ground black pepper
    1 dessertspoon fresh chives, finely chopped
    2 teaspoons butter

Method

Separate the eggs, taking extra care not to allow any yolk into the whites. The whites should be placed in a large clean and dry bowl. The yolks should be placed in a smaller bowl. Beat the egg whites with an electric mixer until soft peaks form. In a separate bowl, lightly beat the egg yolks with a fork and add pepper. Heat the butter in a medium-sized nonstick frying pan and preheat the griller. Gently fold the egg yolk into the whites, along with the mozzarella and chives. Spoon the mixture evenly into the pan and allow it to cook for around 1–2 minutes, or until it begins to set underneath. Remove pan from the hotplate and place it under the griller until the omelette is just set but not overcooked. Use a spatula to carefully loosen the omelette from the pan and fold it in half. Slide onto a serving plate and sprinkle with parmesan cheese and ground black pepper. Serve hot with a grilled tomato on the side.

The above recipe is calculated as 1 serving.

Serving size according to your LBW category:

A ½ serving

B ½ serving + 20 g extra cheese (any variety)

C ½ serving + 40 g extra cheese

D 1 serving

E 1 serving + 20 g extra cheese

F 1 serving + 40 g extra cheese

GRILLED TOMATOES

Ingredients

3 large roma tomatoes

60 g reduced-fat fetta cheese

6 slices shaved, lean ham or prosciutto

1 tablespoon unrefined oil (for cooking)

sea salt

fresh ground black peppercorns

Method

While preheating the griller, cut the tomatoes in half length-wise. Arrange, cut side up, on a nonstick baking tray. Brush lightly with oil and grill for 4–5 minutes. Equally divide slices of fetta and place on top of tomato halves. Sprinkle with sea salt and ground peppercorns, and wrap a slice of ham around each half. Brush with remaining oil and return to the griller for another 3–4 minutes. Serve hot.

The above recipe is calculated as 1 serving.

Serving size according to your LBW category:

A ½ serving

B ½ serving + 1 egg (poached, boiled or scrambled)

C ½ serving + 2 eggs (as above)

D 1 serving

E 1 serving + 1 egg (as above)

F 1 serving + 2 eggs (as above)

OATCAKES

Ingredients

Select ingredient quantities according to your LBW category:

	A	**B**	**C**	**D**	**E**	**F**
quick oats	30 g	40 g	50 g	60 g	70 g	80 g
egg white	2	3	3	4	5	6
whole egg	1	1	2	2	2	3
approved sweetener						
to taste (optional – see pages 121–125)						
fresh or frozen						
mixed berries,						
pureed	50 g	75 g	100 g	125 g	150 g	150 g

Method

Put all ingredients (except berries) into a food processor and blend until thoroughly combined. Preheat a nonstick pan. Brush lightly with cooking oil and add the blended mixture. Pour in enough to cover the bottom of the pan. If you are working with a lot of mixture, cook in batches as you would pancakes. Allow to set and lightly brown underneath, then flip over to cook the other side. Pureed berries may be served hot or cold. Pour berries over the oatcakes and serve immediately.

main meals

BOLOGNAISE WITH A TWIST!

Ingredients

150 g extra-lean beef mince

½ cup onion, finely diced

½ tablespoon unrefined oil (suitable for cooking)

100 g canned pureed tomatoes (no additives)

1 tablespoon tomato paste

½ teaspoon dried oregano

½ teaspoon dried basil

1 clove garlic, crushed (optional)

1 tablespoon parmesan cheese, grated

500 g mixed vegetables (e.g. broccoli, cauliflower, snow peas, button squash, capsicum, cabbage, spinach etc.)

Method

Heat oil in a large nonstick frying pan. Lightly sauté the onion and garlic until softened. Add the meat to the pan and stir until browned. Add the pureed tomatoes, paste and herbs. Bring to the boil. Turn down the heat and cover. Gently simmer for approximately 1 hour. Steam or microwave the mixed vegetables and arrange on a plate. Spoon over the meat sauce and sprinkle with parmesan cheese.

The above recipe is calculated as 1 serving.

Serving size according to your LBW category:

A ½ serving

B ½ serving – with extra vegetables

C ½ serving – with extra vegetables and extra parmesan

D 1 serving

E 1 serving – with extra vegetables

F 1 serving – with extra vegetables and extra parmesan

BURGER MELTS

Ingredients

    200 g extra-lean beef mince
    1 small brown onion, finely diced
    ½ cup grated carrot
    1 tablespoon 'hot' taco sauce (no added sugar)
    ½ teaspoon season-all spice
    1 medium tomato, sliced
    2 tablespoons grated parmesan and mozzarella cheese

Method

In a large mixing bowl combine mince, onion, carrot, sauce and seasoning. Mix together until well combined then form into two equal patties. Refrigerate for 2 hours. Grill the burgers until thoroughly cooked. Place a slice of tomato and half of the cheese on each burger and return to the grill until the cheese has melted. Serve with a green salad.

The above recipe is calculated as 1 serving.

Serving size according to your LBW category:

A ½ serving

B ½ serving + 1 hard-boiled egg in side salad

C 1 serving

D 1 serving + 1 hard-boiled egg in side salad

E 1½ servings

F 1½ servings + 1 hard-boiled egg in side salad

PORK STIR-FRY

Ingredients

Select ingredient quantities according to your LBW category:

	A	B	C	D	E	F
'trim' pork fillets	120 g	150 g	200 g	220 g	250 g	280 g
baby carrots, cut into strips	1	2	3	3	4	4
asparagus spears, halved	3	3	4	4	5	5
red capsicum, cut into strips	1	1	1½	1½	2	2
bok choy, cut lengthwise into quarters	2	2	3	3	4	4
Chinese cabbage, shredded (cups)	1	1	1½	1½	2	2
sugar-free tomato sauce (tablespoons)	2	2	3	3	4	4
light soy sauce	2	2	3	3	4	4
juice of 1 freshly squeezed lemon						

Method

Combine tomato sauce, soy sauce and lemon juice in a shallow bowl. Cut pork into thin strips and add to the sauce. Allow to stand for 30 minutes. Heat a nonstick frying pan or wok. Add pork strips in sauce. Stir-fry until lightly browned, add all vegetables and continue cooking until just tender. Serve.

WARM LAMB AND AVOCADO SALAD

Ingredients
Select ingredient quantities according to your LBW category:

	A	B	C	D	E	F
'trim' lamb fillets	100 g	125 g	150 g	175 g	200 g	225 g
snow peas (pods)	10	10	10	15	15	15
cherry tomatoes						
(small)	8	8	10	12	12	12
rocket (cups)	2	2	3	3	4	4
avocado (2 cm cubes)	4	6	8	8	8	10
yellow or orange						
capsicum, cut into						
strips	½	½	1	1	1	1
Lebanese cucumber,						
julienne	1	1	1	1	1	1
fresh mint leaves for garnish						
balsamic vinegar as dressing						

Method
Prepare all vegetables and arrange on a serving plate. Grill the lamb fillets or dry-fry in a nonstick pan. When cooked, slice lamb into 1.5-cm pieces and arrange over the salad vegetables. Drizzle vinegar over the top and garnish with fresh mint leaves.

SEAFOOD COMBINATION

Ingredients

8 shelled, uncooked prawns, heads removed

100 g firm, boneless fish fillet, cut into 3-cm cubes,
e.g. swordfish, barramundi, tuna or salmon

freshly ground black pepper

4 cups assorted vegetables, e.g. broccoli, capsicum, snow peas,
cabbage, asparagus and carrot

1 tablespoon unrefined olive oil

juice of 1 freshly squeezed lime

juice of 1 freshly squeezed lemon

1 lemon cut into wedges for serving

Method

Prepare prawns and fish. Place in a shallow bowl with combined oil and lemon and lime juice. Allow to marinate for 1–2 hours. Prepare the vegetables, taking care to cut them into similarly sized portions to ensure they are cooked evenly. Heat a nonstick wok or frying pan. Add prawns and fish with any excess marinade. Cook over a high heat for approximately 2 minutes, or until prawns begin to change colour. Add the vegetables to the pan and stir-fry until just tender. Spoon onto serving plates and garnish with freshly ground black pepper and a wedge of lemon.

The above recipe is calculated as 1 serving.

Serving size according to your LBW category:

A ½ serving

B ½ serving + extra vegetables

C ½ serving + 3 extra prawns and extra vegetables

D 1 serving

E 1 serving + extra vegetables

F 1 serving + 3 extra prawns and extra vegetables

TUNA AND COTTAGE DIP

Ingredients

Select ingredient quantities according to your LBW category:

	A	B	C	D	E	F
tuna (tinned)	100 g	120 g	150 g	180 g	200 g	220 g
plain cottage cheese *	50 g	60 g	80 g	100 g	100 g	120 g
mayonnaise * (tablespoon)	1	1	1	1½	2	2
balsamic vinegar (tablespoon)	1	1	1	1½	2	2½
flaxseed oil (teaspoon)	1	1	2	2	2	2

salt and pepper (optional)

Unlimited fresh vegetable sticks for dipping, e.g. carrots, celery, cucumber, green beans or blanched asparagus, broccoli and cauliflower

* see page 139 for information about cheese and page 186 for information about mayonnaise.

Method

In a mixing bowl combine tuna, cheese, mayonnaise, vinegar and oil. Season if desired. Using a fork, mix until thoroughly combined. Spoon into a serving bowl/container and serve with crisp, fresh vegetables for dipping.

GNOCCHI

Ingredients

125 g frozen spinach, defrosted
125 g reduced-fat ricotta cheese
50 g parmesan cheese, shredded
1 egg
freshly ground black pepper
¼ teaspoon nutmeg
1 tablespoon butter, melted

Method

Squeeze moisture out of spinach and chop finely. Combine the spinach, ricotta, half the parmesan, egg, pepper and nutmeg. Mould tablespoons of the mixture into oblongs. Refrigerate for 2 hours. Boil a large pan of water and drop in the gnocchi a few at a time. When they rise, remove with a slotted spoon and transfer to a shallow casserole dish brushed with oil. Drizzle butter over the top, then sprinkle with remaining cheese. Toast under a grill. Serve with a green salad.

The above recipe is calculated as 1 serving.

Serving size according to your LBW category:

A ½ serving

B ½ serving + 1 tablespoon extra grated parmesan

C ½ serving + side salad with 1 dessertspoon of flaxseed oil in dressing

D ½ serving + parmesan and oil (as above)

E 1 serving

F 1 serving + parmesan (as above)

ACCOMPANIMENTS

ASPARAGUS AND PARMESAN

Ingredients

250 g (12 spears) asparagus, woody ends removed

40 g parmesan cheese, freshly shaved

balsamic vinegar

freshly ground black pepper

Method

Brush or spray a preheated, nonstick frying pan with cooking oil. Add the asparagus spears to the pan and cook, turning constantly, until tender. Place asparagus on a serving plate. Drizzle vinegar over the top and garnish with freshly ground black pepper and parmesan shavings.

This makes an ideal accompaniment to lean meat, chicken or fish.

The above recipe is calculated as 1 serving.

Serving size according to your LBW category:

A 1 serving + 100 g protein accompaniment

B 1 serving + 140 g protein accompaniment

C 1 serving + 180 g protein accompaniment

D 1½ servings + 200 g protein accompaniment

E 2 servings + 220 g protein accompaniment

F 2 servings + 250 g protein accompaniment

CAPRESE SALAD

Ingredients

4 roma tomatoes

3 bocconcini, drained

½ cup fresh basil leaves

balsamic vinegar

sea salt

freshly ground black pepper

Method

Slice the bocconcini and tomatoes lengthwise. Arrange the tomato slices on a serving plate and top each with a slice of bocconcini. Arrange the basil leaves over the top and drizzle with balsamic vinegar. Season with freshly ground black pepper and sea salt.

This dish goes well with any chosen protein ... even for breakfast!

The above recipe is calculated as one serving:

Serving size according to your LBW category:

A ½ serving + 80 g protein accompaniment

B ½ serving + 110 g protein accompaniment

C ½ serving + 150 g protein accompaniment

D 1 serving + 150 g protein accompaniment

E 1 serving + 170 g protein accompaniment

F 1 serving + 200 g protein accompaniment

HAWAIIAN SALAD

Ingredients

2 slices of pineapple, 2 cm thick

½ small cantaloupe, skin and seeds removed, cut into slices
   3 cm thick

1 kiwifruit, skin removed and sliced

pulp of 2 small passionfruit

2 thick slices of an extra-large tomato

2 cups mixed salad leaves

ground black pepper

flesh of 1 medium-sized mango, pureed and chilled

Method

Place a slice of tomato in the centre of each plate. Sprinkle with
pepper. Arrange the fruit around the outer rim of the serving
plates. Neatly stack the salad leaves on top of the tomato slice
and pour mango dressing over the top. Serve immediately with
fish/seafood or chicken.

The above recipe is calculated as 1 serving.

Serving size according to your LBW category:

A ½ serving + 130 g protein accompaniment

B ½ serving + 150 g protein accompaniment

C ½ serving + 170 g protein accompaniment

D 1 serving + 170 g protein accompaniment

E 1 serving + 200 g protein accompaniment

F 1 serving + 250 g protein accompaniment

MEDITERRANEAN SALAD

Ingredients

Select ingredient quantities according to your LBW category:

	A	B	C	D	E	F
roma tomato, cut lengthwise into quarters	1	1	1½	1½	2	2
Lebanese cucumber, finely sliced	½	½	1	1	1½	1½
small Spanish (red) onion, cut into thin rings	½	½	1	1	1	1
green capsicum *	¼	¼	½	½	1	1
orange or yellow capsicum *	¼	¼	½	½	1	1
red capsicum *	¼	¼	½	½	1	1
reduced-fat fetta cheese	20 g	25 g	30 g	35 g	40 g	40 g
oregano (fresh or dried)						
balsamic vinegar (tablespoons)	1	1	2	2	3	3
flaxseed oil	10 ml	10 ml	10 ml	10 ml	15 ml	20 ml

juice of 1 freshly squeezed lemon (optional)

* all cut lengthwise into thin strips

Method

Combine all prepared vegetables in a serving bowl. Combine oil
and vinegar (and lemon if included), pour over the vegetables
and toss lightly. Crumble fetta cheese over the top and garnish
with oregano.

ROASTED VEGETABLES

Ingredients

2 slices of pumpkin with skin, 3 cm thick

1 large parsnip, cut into quarters

1 large red capsicum, quartered

1 green capsicum, quartered

1 tablespoon unrefined cooking oil

1 teaspoon sea salt

1 teaspoon ground paprika

Method

Heat the oven to 190°C. Prepare all vegetables. Arrange pumpkin on a baking tray lined with nonstick baking paper. Brush lightly with oil and sprinkle with salt and paprika. Bake for approximately 30 minutes, then add parsnip and capsicum (skin-side up). Brush with oil and sprinkle with seasoning (as above) and return to the oven for 30 minutes. Serve as an accompaniment to lean beef, chicken or fish.

The above recipe is calculated as 1 serving.

Serving size according to your LBW category:

A ½ serving + 80 g protein accompaniment

B ½ serving + 100 g protein accompaniment

C ½ serving + 130 g protein accompaniment

D 1 serving + 130 g protein accompaniment

E 1 serving + 150 g protein accompaniment

F 1 serving + 170 g protein accompaniment

VEGETABLE STIR-FRY

Ingredients

Select ingredient quantities according to your LBW category:

	A	B	C	D	E	F
carrot (small), cut julienne	½	½	1	1	1½	1½
red capsicum, cut lengthwise into thin strips	½	½	1	1	1½	1½
broccoli, small florets	2	2	3	3	4	4
button squash, sliced	50 g	50 g	100 g	100 g	150 g	150 g
snow peas	10	10	10	15	15	15
salt-reduced soy sauce (tablespoons)	1	1½	2	2½	3	3½
freshly squeezed lemon juice (tablespoons)	1	1½	1½	2	2	2½
cold-pressed, unrefined oil (tablespoons) (suitable for cooking)	½	½	1	1	1½	1½

Add any favourite herbs and spices if you prefer extra flavour.

Note: vegetables will cook evenly if they are cut in similar proportions.

Method

Prepare all vegetables. Heat the oil in a large nonstick pan or wok. Place all vegetables in the heated oil and pour over soy and lemon. Lightly toss vegetables until tender, but allow them to remain crunchy. Remove from the pan and serve immediately.

To achieve a desirable balance of nutrition, serve with chicken, steak or fish (see seven-day menu planner). For a vegetarian alternative, you can add tofu to the above recipe, or cook a plain omelette, cut it into thin strips and toss it through the cooked vegetables.

The above-listed quantities are to provide a guideline for each category. You may exceed the vegetable quantity for your category if desired.

VEGGIE-SLAW

Ingredients

Select ingredient quantities according to your LBW category:

	A	B	C	D	E	F
red and green cabbage, shredded (cups)	1	1	1½	1½	2	2
carrot, shredded/ grated (cups)	½	½	1	1	1½	1½
red and yellow capsicum, cut into fine strips (cups)	1	1	1½	1½	2	2
Lebanese cucumber, cut into fine strips	½	½	1	1	1½	1½
homemade* or commercial mayonnaise (tablespoons)	1	1	1½	1½	2	2

juice of 1 freshly squeezed medium-sized lemon

* see page 186

Method

Prepare all above-listed vegetables and combine in a large mixing bowl. In a separate container, combine the mayonnaise and lemon juice. Gradually add cold water until the dressing is diluted to a desired consistency. Pour the dressing over the vegetables and toss until they are evenly coated. Serve as an accompaniment to beef, chicken or fish.

VEGGIE SMASH

Ingredients

Select ingredient quantities according to your LBW category:

	A	B	C	D	E	F
small white or brown onion, finely diced	¼	¼	½	½	1	1
pumpkin (any variety), diced	80 g	80 g	120 g	120 g	150 g	150 g
cauliflower, cut into small florets	50 g	50 g	100 g	100 g	150 g	150 g
cabbage, finely shredded (cups)	½	½	½	1	1	1
almond meal	10 g	10 g	15 g	15 g	20 g	20 g

season-all spice and/or a dash of Tabasco sauce (optional)

Method

Prepare all of the above-listed ingredients. Steam or microwave (without water) the combined vegetables until quite soft. Drain off any excess liquid. Transfer the vegetables to a mixing bowl. Add almond meal, seasoning and Tabasco. Mash together with an electric mixer until thoroughly combined. Form mixture into small, burger-like patties and place on a greased piece of foil. Lightly brown under a preheated grill and serve immediately.

Note: this recipe is structured to serve as an accompaniment to protein. As a vegetarian alternative, you could try melting some grated cheese over the top of the patties prior to grilling.

snacks and desserts

CHEESE PLATTER

Ingredients

Select ingredient quantities according to your LBW category:

	A	B	C	D	E	F
brie	20 g	20 g	30 g	30 g	40 g	50 g
camembert	20 g	20 g	30 g	30 g	40 g	50 g
cheddar, Swiss or edam	20 g	40 g	30 g	50 g	60 g	60 g
apple, cut into quarters then thinly sliced	1 small	1 small	1 medium	1 medium	1 large	1 large
strawberries	6	6	6	6	6	6

Method

Arrange your selection of cheese and fruit on a serving plate. This may be eaten in place of a morning or afternoon snack. If you skip a snack during the day, it may be eaten as dessert.

PARMESAN CRISPS

Ingredients

Select ingredient quantities according to your LBW category:

	A	B	C	D	E	F
grated parmesan cheese (tablespoons)	4	5	6	8	9	10

Method

Form small mounds (equivalent to 1 tablespoon each) on non-stick baking paper. Place under a preheated griller until melted and slightly browned. Remove and allow to cool and become crispy, resembling potato crisps.

Parmesan crisps can be used in place of parmesan cheese in other recipes or can be eaten as a snack with a selection of fresh fruit such as an apple and 10 fresh strawberries.

CHICKEN SANDWICH

Ingredients

    1 skinless chicken fillet, cooked and chilled (150 g raw weight)

    1 tablespoon mashed avocado

    1 tablespoon combined mozzarella and parmesan cheeses, grated

    1 small tomato, sliced

    2 large, crisp cos lettuce leaves, shredded

Method

The chicken breast is taking the place of pita bread. Using a sharp knife, carefully cut the fillet from the thin edge to create a *hinged* opening. Spread the inside of the fillet with avocado, then stuff with cheese, tomato and lettuce. Season to taste.

This is a great midday snack.

The above recipe is calculated as 1 serving.

Serving size according to your LBW category:

A 1 serving

B 1 serving – add a hard-boiled egg to filling

C 1½ servings

D 1½ servings – add a hard-boiled egg to filling

E 2 servings

F 2 servings – add a hard-boiled egg to filling

JELLIED BERRIES

Ingredients

1 cup mixed berries (fresh or frozen)

sugar-free jelly – enough to make up 500 ml

100 g full-cream yoghurt

20 g protein powder (vanilla)

½ teaspoon vanilla essence and 1 dessertspoon approved
sweetener (optional – see pages 121–125)

Method

Make up jelly to 500 ml according to packet instructions. Allow
to cool. Divide the berries into two serving bowls/ramekins with
approximately a 2-cup capacity. Pour the cooled jelly over berries
and refrigerate until set. Mix remaining ingredients together as
'protein yoghurt'. Refrigerate. Serve jellied berries with yoghurt.

This item can be substituted for a midmorning or afternoon snack in the seven-day menu planner. You can skip a
snack through the day and have it as an evening dessert.

The above recipe is calculated as 1 serving.

Serving size according to your LBW category:

A 1 serving

B 1 serving (using 1½ servings of protein yoghurt)

C 1½ servings

D 2 servings

E 2 servings (using 2½ servings of protein yoghurt)

F 2½ servings

FUDGE

Ingredients

    50 g protein powder (see page 142)

    25 g almond meal

    25 g approved sweetener (see pages 121–125)

    25 g plain cocoa powder

    25 g desiccated coconut

    1 rounded tablespoon of hulled tahini paste or nut paste

    cold water

Method

Place all dry ingredients in a large mixing bowl. Add the tahini/nut paste. Using your fingers, rub the paste into the dry ingredients until it is evenly distributed. Gradually begin to add water in very small amounts. Continue to knead the mixture until it becomes a stiff 'dough'. Be sure not to add too much water as the mixture will become too sticky and hard to handle. Place the mixture on a clean, dry surface and mould with your hands until it forms a log. Cover it completely with foil and refrigerate for a few hours, or overnight. To serve, cut from the end into ten 2 cm rounds.

One slice is calculated as 1 serving. Serving size category is indicated in the seven-day menu planner.

miscellaneous

MAYONNAISE

Ingredients

2 egg yolks

2 teaspoons Dijon mustard

2 teaspoons freshly squeezed lemon juice

1 cup unrefined oil *

salt and pepper

*Your choice will depend on personal taste. I recommend
flaxseed, sunflower or cold-pressed olive oil.

Method

Place egg yolk, lemon juice and mustard in a blender and
process until thoroughly combined and creamy (approximately
30 seconds). Continue mixing at a low speed while gradually
pouring in the oil. Stir in lemon juice and season with a sprinkle of salt and pepper.

If you prefer a sweeter taste, you may try adding a teaspoon
of approved sweetener (see pages 121–125).

appendix

MEDICAL CASE STUDIES

I am grateful to Dr Bruce Farnsworth for supplying details of the following case studies. Dr Farnsworth is a Sydney-based consultant gynaecologist who specialises in hormone problems, bladder problems and bleeding problems and who uses a medically supervised version of my diet and exercise program to achieve great results for many patients.

Case 1: Bronwyn

Bronwyn was a 37-year-old housewife who presented to Dr Farnsworth with symptoms suggesting hormonal imbalance, including heavy periods with clots, breast tenderness, fluid retention, abdominal bloating, headaches and weight gain. At 102 kg, Bronwyn had steadily gained weight following the birth of her only child. She also suffered from decreased libido, sleep problems and sugar cravings. Blood tests revealed that Bronwyn had an elevated level of fasting serum insulin as well as abnormal cholesterol and triglyceride levels.

Bronwyn achieved immediate results on the diet part of the program. Within a week her bloating and sugar cravings had disappeared. Initially Bronwyn did have some headaches and feelings of tiredness, but these may have been due to a concurrent sinus infection.

By week five Bronwyn had lost 7 kg. Enthusiastic about starting the exercise component of the program, she began regular visits to the gym. At the conclusion of her formal ten-week program Bronwyn had lost a total of 10 kg. Her general health had

improved considerably and repeated blood tests confirmed the
following improvements:

	BEFORE	AFTER
Cholesterol	7.4	6.1
Triglycerides	3.21	1.06
Insulin	19.2	12.6

In addition, her ratio of 'good' cholesterol to 'bad' cholesterol
had improved.

Bronwyn is determined to stick to her program and hopes
eventually to reach her goal weight and see her cholesterol
reduced to a normal level.

Case 2: Cathy

Cathy is a 41-year-old supermarket employee who presented with
heavy periods, weight gain, abdominal bloating, tiredness and dry
skin. She had steadily gained weight since her two children had
been delivered by caesarean section, after which she had had her
tubes tied. She did not suffer from sugar cravings, fluid retention
or headaches.

Investigations revealed that Cathy had large fibroids in her
uterus. She eventually had a partial hysterectomy, in which only
the fibroids were removed. After the operation, a diet and lifestyle
program was suggested to help her lose weight and improve her
general health.

'I found this diet very simple to follow,' says Cathy. 'The meals
are easy to prepare and are very nutritious. The meals that you can
eat are no different to your normal meals.'

Cathy found that the whole family would eat the meals without complaint. 'Before starting the program I weighed 110 kg. My weight is now 89 kg, so after just seven months I have lost 21 kg and I feel fantastic. At 110 kg I was suffering from high blood pressure, high cholesterol, high blood sugar, heart palpitations and low energy. All of these symptoms have been reduced and I cannot get over the difference that the weight loss has made to me. Over the last few months the rate of weight loss has slowed but I continue to stick with the diet and I am still losing weight. My husband has also been on the diet and has lost about 15 kg. He has found that he can eat meals that he likes and lose weight just by being sensible. I would recommend this diet to anyone.'

Cathy's response has been spectacular. Her cholesterol levels are now normal and she has started to exercise regularly.

Case 3: Jenny

Jenny is a 30-year-old office worker who presented to Dr Farnsworth with period problems and abdominal pain. She had been diagnosed and investigated for chronic fatigue syndrome for four years. Jenny suffered from breast tenderness, abdominal bloating, migraines, tiredness, premenstrual symptoms and sleep problems. She had severe sugar cravings, hypoglycaemic episodes, food allergies and yeast infections.

Jenny has had an excellent response to treatment. In the first two months she has lost over 10 kg. Her cholesterol has dropped from 6.5 to 5.1. She has also noticed a dramatic improvement in her symptoms. She is determined to continue losing weight, do more exercise and improve her general health.

Case 4: Ellen

Ellen is a 45-year-old who presented to her local doctor with left-sided pelvic pain and back pain. The suspected diagnosis was irritable bowel syndrome. Her colonoscopy proved to be normal but a pelvic ultrasound revealed ovarian cysts and Ellen was referred to Dr Farnsworth. A laparoscopic partial oophorectomy (removal of the ovaries) was performed and Ellen was given the option of trying to use diet to reduce insulin levels and suppress ovarian cyst formation.

'I began the diet in March 2000. I found it easy to follow and soon my weight began to fall off. I noticed that my pains had settled down, my blood results were amazing, people were telling me I looked great and I felt fantastic. I've lost 10 kg in the past five months.'

Ellen's blood test results are listed below:

	BEFORE	AFTER TWO MONTHS
Fasting insulin	23	8
Cholesterol	6.5	4.9
Glucose	5.6	5.1

The dramatic results that Ellen achieved in the first two months of treatment were a wonderful incentive for her to go on to achieve long-term changes in her health and lifestyle.

bibliography

Australian Bureau of Statistics 1995, *How Australians Measure Up*, Cat. No. 4359.0, ABS, Canberra.

Bernstein, J., et al. 1977, 'Depression of lymphocyte transformation following oral glucose ingestion', *American Journal of Clinical Nutrition*, 30:613.

Chaitow, Leon 2000, *Antioxidants and Ageing*, HealthWorld Online: Life Extension.

Connor, W.E. 1999, 'A-linolenic acid in health and disease', *American Journal of Clinical Nutrition*, 69:827–828.

Dumonteil, E., Magnan, C., Ritz-Lasar, B., Ktorza, A., Meda, P., Philippe, J. 2000, *Endocrinology*, 141 (1): 174–80.

Harman, D. 1999–2000, 'The free-radical theory of ageing: Part 2 – Calorie restriction, free radicals and new research', *Encyclopaedia Britannica.com*.

Knox, L. S., Crosby, L. O., Feurer, I. D., et al. 1983, 'Energy expenditure in malnourished cancer patients', *Annual-Surgery*, 197:152–61.

Lee, A. T., et al. 1992, 'Role of glycation in ageing', *Annals of the New York Academy of Sciences*, 663:63–70.

Life Extension – Disease Prevention and Treatment 2000, 3rd edition, Life Extension Media, USA.

McDonald, R. B. 1995, 'Influence of dietary sucrose on

biological ageing', *American Journal of Clinical Nutrition*, 62 (suppl.):284S–93S.

National Research Council, USA 1996, *Recommended Dietary Allowances*, 11th edition, National Academy Press.

Ravussin E., Lillioja S., Anderson T. E., Christin L., Bogardus C. 1986, 'Determinants of 24 hour energy expenditure in man', *Journal of Clinical Investigation*, 78:1568–78.

Sarjeant, D., E. & K. 1999, *Hard to Swallow: the truth about food additives*, Alive Books, Vancouver.

Segal K. R., Albu J., Chun A., Edano A., Legaspi B., Pi-Sunyer F. X. 1992, 'Independent effects of obesity and insulin resistance on postprandial thermogenesis in men', *Journal of Clinical Investigation*, 89:824–33.

Segal K. R., Gutin B., Nyman A. M., Pi-Sunyer F. X. 1985, 'Thermic effect of food at rest, during exercise, and after exercise in lean and obese men of similar body weight', *Journal of Clinical Investigation*, 76:1107–12.

Serraino, M., et al. 1991, 'The effect of flaxseed supplementation on early risk markers for mammary carcinogenesis', *Cancer Letters*, 60:135-142.

Splenda Food Additive Petition 7A3987, pp. 623–731.

White, J. W., Wolraich, M. 1995, 'Effect of sugar on behaviour and mental performance', *The American Journal of Clinical Nutrition*, 62 (suppl.):242S–9S.

glossary

Ab-roller An exercise apparatus offering neck support and designed to enable abdominal exercise to be undertaken correctly.

Absorption The process by which nutrients from our food are taken up by our digestive tract and passed into the bloodstream for use.

Adipose Masses of fat cells that form a layer of body fat beneath the skin.

Adrenal glands Glands that produce corticosteroid hormones in response to stress and trauma.

Allergic reaction A reaction of body tissue to a specific substance.

Altered fats Dietary fats that have been exposed to heat, light and oxygen during processing and as a result have had their original molecular structure changed, often rendering them harmful to health.

Amino acids The building blocks of proteins; there are over 20 known amino acids present in nature.

Anaemia A reduction in the quantity of oxygen-carrying haemoglobin (red blood cells) in the blood; causes include iron deficiency and blood loss.

Anti-ageing Attempting to slow down the degenerative process of ageing – preventative nutrition and life extension.

Anti-oxidant A substance that combats or neutralises free radicals before our body cells are damaged excessively.

Artificial sweetener In the context of this book, artificial sweetening substances are modified, calorie-reduced sweetening substances (see Chapter 11), as opposed to high-carbohydrate sugar derivatives that create a greater insulin response when ingested.

Balanced meal/diet A meal or dietary plan that includes a balance of essential nutrients in the correct ratios.

Basal metabolic rate (BMR) The minimal amount of energy expended by the body to maintain vital processes such as respiration, circulation and digestion.

Bioflavonoids A new class of vitamin compound found in all fruits and vegetables. Research into flavonoids is still in its infancy but it is believed they may offer protection against cancer and other degenerative diseases.

Biological age This is the age of our body according to our physical state, as opposed to our age in years since our birth date.

Blood-sugar estimation An important factor in detecting many diseases.

Blood-sugar level The concentration of glucose (sugar) in the blood.

Body composition The ratio of fat to lean tissue in your body.

Body fat Fat accumulated in 'storage tanks' (fat cells) in the body.

Body-fat distribution Refers to the location, or placement, of fat cells in an individual's body.

Botulin The toxin causing botulism (serious food poisoning).

Botulinus The bacterium *Clostridium botulinum*, which thrives in improperly stored and preserved foods and forms botulin.

Calorie (cal) An Imperial unit of measurement used to indicate the energy value of food.

Carbohydrates Carbohydrates are manufactured by plants. This term covers a large group of both processed and unprocessed varieties, including sugars, grains, fruits and vegetables.

Cardiovascular exercise This is exercise that increases the heart rate, circulation and rate of breathing, eventually improving cardiovascular capacity.

Carnivore One who consumes meat.

Cellulite A visibly uneven, lumpy form of fat beneath the skin, usually found on the hips and buttocks of females due to an excess accumulation of fat cells in a concentrated area.

Chronological age Our age according to our birth date (*see* Biological age).

Cold pressed Usually refers to the process of extracting oils from their source – the term 'cold pressed' indicates the absence of damaging heat often used in extraction.

Commercial products Mass-produced, processed, packaged food products.

Deficiency disease Any disease caused by the lack of an essential nutrient in the diet.

Degenerative diseases Diseases that can cause permanent deterioration of the tissues, such as osteoarthritis, arteriosclerosis and cancer, among hundreds of others.

Diabetes A disorder of carbohydrate metabolism in which sugars in the body are not processed effectively due to a lack of insulin, or insulin resistance. Insulin resistance is usually developed later in life due to incorrect dietary habits, creating an excessive demand on insulin response to sugars.

Digestion The process in which the food we eat is broken down into a form that can be absorbed and used by the body.

DNA The genetic material in nearly all living things that passes on genetic information when cells naturally divide and replicate themselves.

Empty calories Processed foods that contain a high level of calories yet are devoid of essential nutritional value.

Energy balance A balance between the energy we eat and the energy we require, or burn off.

Energy burn The utilisation of calories (energy) by the body, whether in the form of ingested foods, glycogen (blood sugar) or the release of stored fats.

Enzyme A protein formed in living cells and assisting in numerous chemical processes within the body.

Essential fats Fats that must be taken in through the diet. They cannot be assimilated in the body as some nutrients can be.

Fat cells The 'storage tanks' in which we store excess body fat for reserve energy and insulation.

Fat-soluble substance A substance that is only dissolved or absorbed in the presence of fat.

Fibre Any of several indigestible carbohydrates that make up the 'roughage' of plant material.

Fortified product A food product that has had selected nutrients added.

Free radicals Highly unstable particles that are produced as a normal part of metabolism. Excessive amounts can be harmful to cells and DNA and require the neutralising action of anti-oxidants. The production of excessive amounts can be triggered by such things as radiation, UV exposure, smoke and pollution.

Genetically modified organism (GMO) An organism that has been genetically manipulated to create 'super-foods'. Can improve crop harvests, the shelf life of food products etc.

Genetics The science of inheritance of our physical characteristics and personality traits.

Glucagon A hormone released by the pancreas to increase blood-sugar levels.

Glucose A simple sugar.

Glycogen The form in which glucose is stored in the body.

Haemoglobin A substance contained within red blood cells that transports oxygen in the body. Haemoglobin is responsible for the red colour of blood.

High-density lipoprotein (HDL) The so-called 'good' cholesterol, HDLs carry excess cholesterol from the cells to the liver.

Hormones Potent substances produced by the body and carried to organs and tissues to act upon or modify their structure or function. Some examples of hormones are corticosteroids, growth hormone, oestrogen and testosterone.

Hydrogenation A method of food processing in which hydrogen is introduced (as in margarine) to create a solid fat.

Hyper- Excessive, abnormally increased.

Hyperglycaemia Excessively high blood-sugar levels.

Hypo- Abnormally low, decreased.

Hypoglycaemia Low blood-sugar levels.

Immune system The mechanism that protects the body against invading bacteria and disease.

Immunosuppression Suppression of the immune system, reducing the body's defences against invading disease and bacteria.

Insulin A hormone important for regulating the amount of sugar (glucose) present in the blood.

Intestinal flora/bacteria Bacteria normally present in the digestive tract.

Kilojoule (kj) A metric unit of measure used to indicate the energy value of food.

Lean body weight (LBW) LBW refers to the composition of your body. It is the weight of your body excluding stored body fat and comprises such things as muscle, organs, blood and bones.

Lipolysis The process by which fats (lipids) are broken down into fatty acids by the enzyme lipase.

Liposuction A cosmetic surgical procedure in which fat is literally sucked from beneath the skin.

Low-density lipoprotein (LDL) The so-called 'bad cholesterol', LDLs are responsible for carrying cholesterol via the bloodstream to the cells.

Macronutrients The major dietary nutrients – protein, carbohydrates and fats.

Malabsorption A digestive disorder in which nutrients are not absorbed and used effectively.

Malnutrition The condition of a person who does not receive all essential nutrients in appropriate proportions.

Medicine ball A heavy ball available in various weights and used in a variety of exercises.

Metabolism The chemical and physical changes that take place within the body and enable it to continue to function and grow.

Multivitamin/mineral This refers to a supplementary form of combined and balanced vitamins and minerals taken in addition to a balanced diet to prevent nutritional deficiencies.

Mutated gene A gene that has had its structure (DNA) changed.

Nutrient Needed by the body to maintain life and health.

Organic Derived from matter of either animal or plant origin. In farming, the term 'organic' refers to the absence of artificial fertilisers and pesticides in production.

Oxidise To combine with oxygen.

Processed food Food that has been refined and altered so that the final product is nutritionally inferior to the food from which it was made.

Protein Protein is composed of a combination of amino acids and is important in the functioning of enzymes and hormones. It is responsible for forming essential structural material such as muscles, tissues and organs and is obtained from the diet.

Rancid Stale, or 'off'.

'Real' food Unprocessed food in its natural, or 'whole', state.

Recommended dietary allowance/intake Government-set standard of nutrients necessary for the average 'healthy' person to prevent disease.

Refined foods Foods that have been processed and have, therefore, lost some of their nutritional value.

Resistance training Exercise utilising weights.

Speed ball A small ball mounted on the wall with a mounting board. It's commonly used in boxing training for improving hand–eye coordination and agility.

Supplements Nutrients taken in a concentrated form as a tablet, capsule, powder or liquid.

Swiss ball A large, inflatable ball commonly used by gymnasiums and physiotherapists for stretching, rehabilitation and general exercise.

Trans-fatty acids (TFAs) Harmful fats that have been structurally altered by various processing methods.

Triglycerides The form in which fats are stored in the body's fat tissues.

Vegan A person who eats no meat or other animal products.

Vegetarian A person who eats no meat or fish but may consume dairy products and eggs.

Vitamin An organic compound present in food and essential for normal growth and metabolism.

Water soluble A substance that is only dissolved or absorbed in the presence of water.

Weight-bearing exercise Exercise utilising resistance/weights.

Whole foods Foods in their natural, unprocessed state, with nutrients and fibre intact.

Yo-yo dieting Calories are restricted for as long as willpower can be sustained. When willpower diminishes, 'normal' eating resumes and weight is regained with a vengeance.

index